*We cannot change the cards we are dealt,
just how we play the hand.*
Randy Pausch

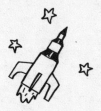

A lot of professors give talks called 'the Last Lecture' reflecting
on what matters most to them and what they'd like to pass on.
In September 2007 computer science professor Randy Pausch
delivered a last lecture called 'Really Achieving Your Childhood
Dreams'. Ironically, it really was his last lecture, as this youthful,
energetic and cheerful man had just been diagnosed with
pancreatic cancer and had only months to live.

Randy's lecture about the joy of life – his legacy to his three
young children – has become a phenomenon, as has this
book written on the same principles, celebrating the dreams
we all try to make a reality.

The Last Lecture is an inspirational and heart-warming book
about living, *not* dying. It should change your life.

Because *'time is all you have… and you may find one day that
you have less time than you think.'*

The
LAST
LECTURE

lessons in living

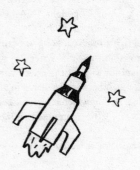

Randy Pausch

Professor, Carnegie Mellon

with Jeffrey Zaslow

HODDER

First published in Great Britain in 2008 by Hodder & Stoughton
An Hachette UK company
Published by arrangement with Hyperion

First published in paperback in 2010

3

A CIP catalogue record for this title is available from the British Library.

ISBN 978 0340 978504

Typeset in Adobe Garamond

Printed and bound in the UK by CPI Mackays, Chatham ME5 8TD

Hodder & Stoughton policy is to use papers that are natural, renewable
and recyclable products and made from wood grown in sustainable
forests. The logging and manufacturing processes are expected to
conform to the environmental regulations of the country of origin.

Hodder & Stoughton Ltd
338 Euston Road
London NW1 3BH

www.hodder.co.uk

With thanks to my parents who allowed me to dream,
and with hopes for the dreams my children will have.

Contents

Introduction

I HAVE AN engineering problem.

While for the most part I'm in terrific physical shape, I have ten tumors in my liver and I have only a few months left to live.

I am a father of three young children, and married to the woman of my dreams. While I could easily feel sorry for myself, that wouldn't do them, or me, any good.

So, how to spend my very limited time?

The obvious part is being with, and taking care of, my family. While I still can, I embrace every moment with them, and do the logistical things necessary to ease their path into a life without me.

The less obvious part is how to teach my children what I would have taught them over the next twenty years. They are too young now to have those conversations. All parents want to teach their children right from wrong, what we think is important, and how to deal with the challenges life will bring. We also want them to know some stories from our own lives, often as a way to teach them how to lead theirs. My desire to do that led me to give a "last lecture" at Carnegie Mellon University.

These lectures are routinely videotaped. I knew what I was doing that day. Under the ruse of giving an academic lecture, I was trying to put myself in a bottle that would one day wash up on the beach for my children. If I were a painter, I would have painted for them. If I were a musician, I would have composed music. But I am a lecturer. So I lectured.

I lectured about the joy of life, about how much I appreciated life, even with so little of my own left. I talked about honesty, integrity, gratitude, and other things I hold dear. And I tried very hard not to be boring.

This book is a way for me to continue what I began on stage. Because time is precious, and I want to spend all that I can with my kids, I asked Jeffrey Zaslow for help. Each day, I ride my bike around my neighborhood, getting exercise crucial for my health. On fifty-three long bike rides, I spoke to Jeff on my cell-phone headset. He then spent countless hours helping to turn my stories—I suppose we could call them fifty-three "lectures"—into the book that follows.

We knew right from the start: None of this is a replacement for a living parent. But engineering isn't about perfect solutions; it's about doing the best you can with limited resources. Both the lecture and this book are my attempts to do exactly that.

I

THE LAST
LECTURE

I

An Injured Lion
Still Wants to Roar

———————

A LOT OF professors give talks titled "The Last Lecture." Maybe you've seen one.

It has become a common exercise on college campuses. Professors are asked to consider their demise and to ruminate on what matters most to them. And while they speak, audiences can't help but mull the same question: What wisdom would we impart to the world if we knew it was our last chance? If we had to vanish tomorrow, what would we want as our legacy?

For years, Carnegie Mellon had a "Last Lecture Series." But by the time organizers got around to asking me to do it, they'd renamed their series "Journeys," asking selected professors "to offer reflections on their personal and professional journeys." It wasn't the most exciting description, but I agreed to go with it. I was given the September slot.

At the time, I already had been diagnosed with pancreatic cancer, but I was optimistic. Maybe I'd be among the lucky ones who'd survive.

While I went through treatment, those running the lecture series kept sending me emails. "What will you be talking about?" they asked. "Please provide an abstract." There's a formality in academia that can't be ignored, even if a man is busy with other things, like trying not to die. By mid-August, I was told that a poster for the lecture had to be printed, so I'd have to decide on a topic.

That very week, however, I got the news: My most recent treatment hadn't worked. I had just months to live.

I knew I could cancel the lecture. Everyone would understand. Suddenly, there were so many other things to be done. I had to deal with my own grief and the sadness of those who loved me. I had to throw myself into getting my family's affairs in order. And yet, despite everything, I couldn't shake the idea of giving the talk. I was energized by the idea of delivering a last lecture that really was a last lecture. What could I say? How would it be received? Could I even get through it?

"They'll let me back out," I told my wife, Jai, "but I really want to do it."

Jai (pronounced "Jay") had always been my cheerleader. When I was enthusiastic, so was she. But she was leery of this whole last-lecture idea. We had just moved from Pittsburgh to Southeastern Virginia so that after my death, Jai and the kids could be near her family. Jai felt that I ought to be spending my precious time with our kids, or unpacking our new house, rather than devoting my hours to writing the lecture and then traveling back to Pittsburgh to deliver it.

"Call me selfish," Jai told me. "But I want all of you. Any

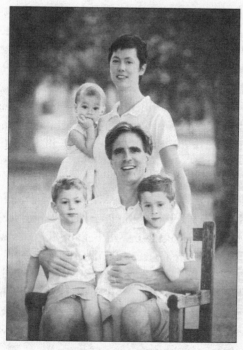

Logan, Chloe, Jai, myself, and Dylan.

time you'll spend working on this lecture is lost time, because it's time away from the kids and from me."

I understood where she was coming from. From the time I'd gotten sick, I had made a pledge to myself to defer to Jai and honor her wishes. I saw it as my mission to do all I could to lessen the burdens in her life brought on by my illness.

That's why I spent many of my waking hours making arrangements for my family's future without me. Still, I couldn't let go of my urge to give this last lecture.

Throughout my academic career, I'd given some pretty good talks. But being considered the best speaker in a computer science department is like being known as the tallest of the Seven Dwarfs. And right then, I had the feeling that I had more in me, that if I gave it my all, I might be able to offer people something special. "Wisdom" is a strong word, but maybe that was it.

Jai still wasn't happy about it. We eventually took the issue to Michele Reiss, the psychotherapist we'd begun seeing a few months earlier. She specializes in helping families when one member is confronting a terminal illness.

"I know Randy," Jai told Dr. Reiss. "He's a workaholic. I know just what he'll be like when he starts putting the lecture together. It'll be all-consuming." The lecture, she argued, would be an unnecessary diversion from the overwhelming issues we were grappling with in our lives.

Another matter upsetting Jai: To give the talk as scheduled, I would have to fly to Pittsburgh the day before, which was Jai's forty-first birthday. "This is my last birthday we'll celebrate together," she told me. "You're actually going to leave me on my birthday?"

Certainly, the thought of leaving Jai that day was painful to me. And yet, I couldn't let go of the idea of the lecture. I had come to see it as the last moment of my career, as a way to say goodbye to my "work family." I also found myself fantasizing about giving a last lecture that would be the oratorical equivalent of a retiring baseball slugger driving one last ball into the upper deck. I *had* always liked the final scene in *The Natural*, when the aging, bleeding ballplayer Roy Hobbs miraculously hits that towering home run.

Dr. Reiss listened to Jai and to me. In Jai, she said, she saw a strong, loving woman who had intended to spend decades building a full life with a husband, raising children to adulthood. Now our lives together had to be squeezed into a few months. In me, Dr. Reiss saw a man not yet ready to fully retreat to his home life, and certainly not yet ready to climb into his deathbed. "This lecture will be the last time many people I care about will see me in the flesh," I told her flatly. "I have a chance here to really think about what matters most to me, to cement how people will remember me, and to do whatever good I can on the way out."

More than once, Dr. Reiss had watched Jai and me sit together on her office couch, holding tightly to each other, both of us in tears. She told us she could see the great respect between us, and she was often viscerally moved by our commitment to getting our final time together right. But she said it wasn't her role to weigh in on whether or not I gave the lecture. "You'll have to decide that on your own," she said, and encouraged us to really listen to each other, so we could make the right decision for both of us.

Given Jai's reticence, I knew I had to look honestly at my motivations. Why was this talk so important to me? Was it a way to remind me and everyone else that I was still very much alive? To prove I still had the fortitude to perform? Was it a limelight-lover's urge to show off one last time? The answer was yes on all fronts. "An injured lion wants to know if he can still roar," I told Jai. "It's about dignity and self-esteem, which isn't quite the same as vanity."

There was something else at work here, too. I had started to view the talk as a vehicle for me to ride into the future I would never see.

I reminded Jai of the kids' ages: five, two and one. "Look," I said. "At five, I suppose that Dylan will grow up to have a few memories of me. But how much will he really remember? What do you and I even remember from when we were five? Will Dylan remember how I played with him, or what he and I laughed about? It may be hazy at best.

"And how about Logan and Chloe? They may have no memories at all. Nothing. Especially Chloe. And I can tell you this: When the kids are older, they're going to go through this phase where they absolutely, achingly need to know: 'Who was my dad? What was he like?' This lecture could help give them an answer to that." I told Jai I'd make sure Carnegie Mellon would record the lecture. "I'll get you a DVD. When the kids are older, you can show it to them. It'll help them understand who I was and what I cared about."

Jai heard me out, then asked the obvious question. "If you have things you want to say to the kids, or advice you want to give them, why not just put a video camera on a tripod and tape it here in the living room?"

Maybe she had me there. Or maybe not. Like that lion in the jungle, my natural habitat was still on a college campus, in front of students. "One thing I've learned," I told Jai, "is that when parents tell children things, it doesn't hurt to get some external validation. If I can get an audience to laugh and clap at the right time, maybe that would add gravitas to what I'm telling the kids."

Jai smiled at me, her dying showman, and finally relented. She knew I'd been yearning to find ways to leave a legacy for the kids. OK. Perhaps this lecture could be an avenue for that.

And so, with Jai's green light, I had a challenge before me. How could I turn this academic talk into something that would resonate with our kids a decade or more up the road?

I knew for sure that I didn't want the lecture to focus on my cancer. My medical saga was what it was, and I'd already been over it and over it. I had little interest in giving a discourse on, say, my insights into how I coped with the disease, or how it gave me new perspectives. Many people might expect the talk to be about dying. But it had to be about *living*.

* * *

"What makes me unique?"

That was the question I felt compelled to address. Maybe answering that would help me figure out what to say. I was sitting with Jai in a doctor's waiting room at Johns Hopkins, awaiting yet another pathology report, and I was bouncing my thoughts off her.

"Cancer doesn't make me unique," I said. There was no

arguing that. More than 37,000 Americans a year are diagnosed with pancreatic cancer alone.

I thought hard about how I defined myself: as a teacher, a computer scientist, a husband, a father, a son, a friend, a brother, a mentor to my students. Those were all roles I valued. But did any of those roles really set me apart?

Though I've always had a healthy sense of self, I knew this lecture needed more than just bravado. I asked myself: "What do I, alone, truly have to offer?"

And then, there in that waiting room, I suddenly knew exactly what it was. It came to me in a flash: Whatever my accomplishments, all of the things I loved were rooted in the dreams and goals I had as a child . . . and in the ways I had managed to fulfill almost all of them. My uniqueness, I realized, came in the specifics of all the dreams—from incredibly meaningful to decidedly quirky—that defined my forty-six years of life. Sitting there, I knew that despite the cancer, I truly believed I was a lucky man because I had lived out these dreams. And I had lived out my dreams, in great measure, because of things I was taught by all sorts of extraordinary people along the way. If I was able to tell my story with the passion I felt, my lecture might help others find a path to fulfilling their own dreams.

I had my laptop with me in that waiting room, and fueled by this epiphany, I quickly tapped out an email to the lecture organizers. I told them I finally had a title for them. "My apologies for the delay," I wrote. "Let's call it: 'Really Achieving Your Childhood Dreams.'"

2

My Life in a Laptop

H OW, EXACTLY, do you catalogue your childhood dreams? How do you get other people to reconnect with theirs? As a scientist, these weren't the questions I typically struggled with.

For four days, I sat at my computer in our new home in Virginia, scanning slides and photos as I built a PowerPoint presentation. I've always been a visual thinker, so I knew the talk would have no text—no word script. But I amassed 300 images of my family, students and colleagues, along with dozens of offbeat illustrations that could make a point about childhood dreams. I put a few words on certain slides—bits of advice, sayings. Once I was on stage, those were supposed to remind me what to say.

As I worked on the talk, I'd rise from my chair every ninety minutes or so to interact with the kids. Jai saw me trying to remain engaged in family life, but she still thought I was spending way too much time on the talk, especially since we'd just arrived in the new house. She, naturally, wanted me to deal with the boxes piled all over our house.

At first, Jai didn't plan to attend the lecture. She felt she needed to stay in Virginia with the kids to deal with the dozens of things that had to get done in the wake of our move. I kept saying, "I want you there." The truth was, I desperately needed her there. And so she eventually agreed to fly to Pittsburgh on the morning of the talk.

I had to get to Pittsburgh a day early, however, so at 1:30 p.m. on September 17, the day Jai turned forty-one, I kissed her and the kids goodbye, and drove to the airport. We had celebrated her birthday the day before with a small party at her brother's house. Still, my departure was an unpleasant reminder for Jai that she'd now be without me for this birthday and all the birthdays to come.

I landed in Pittsburgh and was met at the airport by my friend Steve Seabolt, who'd flown in from San Francisco. We had bonded years earlier, when I did a sabbatical at Electronic Arts, the video-game maker where Steve is an executive. We'd become as close as brothers.

Steve and I embraced, hired a rental car, and drove off together, trading gallows humor. Steve said he'd just been to the dentist, and I bragged that I didn't need to go to the dentist anymore.

We pulled into a local diner to eat, and I put my laptop on the table. I flashed quickly through my slides, now trimmed to 280. "It's still way too long," Steve told me. "Everyone will be dead by the time you're through with the presentation."

The waitress, a pregnant woman in her thirties with dishwater-blond hair, came to our table just as a photo of my children was on the screen. "Cute kids," she said, and asked for their names. I told her: "That's Dylan, Logan, Chloe . . ." The waitress said her daughter's name was Chloe, and we both smiled at the coincidence. Steve and I kept going through the PowerPoint, with Steve helping me focus.

When the waitress brought our meals, I congratulated her on her pregnancy. "You must be overjoyed," I said.

"Not exactly," she responded. "It was an accident."

As she walked away, I couldn't help but be struck by her frankness. Her casual remark was a reminder about the accidental elements that play into both our arrival into life . . . and our departure into death. Here was a woman, having a child by accident that she surely would come to love. As for me, through the accident of cancer I'd be leaving three children to grow up without my love.

An hour later, alone in my room at the hotel, my kids remained in my head as I continued to cut and rearrange images from the talk. The wireless internet access in the room was spotty, which was exasperating because I was still combing the Web, looking for images. Making matters worse, I was starting to feel the effects of the chemo treatment I'd received days before. I had cramps, nausea and diarrhea.

I worked until midnight, fell asleep, and then woke up at 5 a.m. in a panic. A part of me doubted that my talk would work at all. I thought to myself: "This is exactly what you get when you try to tell your whole life story in an hour!"

I kept tinkering, rethinking, reorganizing. By 11 a.m., I felt I had a better narrative arc; maybe it would work. I showered, got dressed. At noon, Jai arrived from the airport and joined me and Steve for lunch. It was a solemn conversation, with Steve vowing to help look after Jai and the kids.

At 1:30 p.m., the computer lab on campus where I spent much of my life was dedicated in my honor; I watched the unveiling of my name over the door. At 2:15 p.m., I was in my office, feeling awful again—completely exhausted, sick from the chemo, and wondering if I'd have to go on stage wearing the adult diaper I'd brought as a precaution.

Steve told me I should lie down on my office couch for a while, and I did, but I kept my laptop on my belly so I could continue to fiddle. I cut another sixty slides.

At 3:30 p.m., a few people had already begun lining up for my talk. At 4 p.m., I roused myself off the couch and started gathering my props for the walk across campus to the lecture hall. In less than an hour, I'd have to be on the stage.

3

The Elephant in the Room

JAI WAS already in the hall—an unexpected full house of 400—and as I hopped on stage to check out the podium and get organized, she could see how nervous I was. While I busied myself arranging my props, Jai noticed that I was making eye contact with almost no one. She thought that I couldn't bring myself to look into the crowd, knowing I might see a friend or former student, and I'd be too overwhelmed by the emotion of that eye contact.

There was a rustling in the audience as I got myself ready. For those who came to see just what a man dying of pancreatic cancer looked like, surely there were questions: Was that my real hair? (Yes, I kept all my hair through chemotherapy.) Would they be able to sense how close to death I was as I spoke? (My answer: "Just watch!")

Even with the talk only minutes away, I continued puttering at the podium, deleting some slides, rearranging others. I was still working at it when I was given the signal. "We're ready to go," someone told me.

*   *   *

I wasn't in a suit. I wore no tie. I wasn't going to get up there in some professorial tweed jacket with leather elbow patches. Instead, I had chosen to give my lecture wearing the most appropriate childhood-dream garb I could find in my closet.

Granted, at first glance I looked like the guy who'd take your order at a fast-food drive-through. But actually, the logo on my short-sleeved polo shirt was an emblem of honor because it's the one worn by Walt Disney Imagineers—the artists, writers and engineers who create theme-park fantasies. In 1995, I spent a six-month sabbatical as an Imagineer. It was a highlight of my life, the fulfillment of a childhood dream. That's why I was also wearing the oval "Randy" name badge given to me when I worked at Disney. I was paying tribute to that life experience, and to Walt Disney himself, who famously had said, "If you can dream it, you can do it."

I thanked the audience for coming, cracked a few jokes, and then I said: "In case there's anybody who wandered in and doesn't know the back story, my dad always taught me that when there's an elephant in the room, introduce it. If you look at my CT scans, there are approximately ten tumors in my liver, and the doctors told me I have three to six months of good health left. That was a month ago, so you can do the math."

I flashed a giant image of the CT scans of my liver onto the screen. The slide was headlined "The Elephant in the Room," and I had helpfully inserted red arrows pointing to each of the individual tumors.

I let the slide linger, so the audience could follow the arrows and count my tumors. "All right," I said. "That is what it is. We can't change it. We just have to decide how we'll respond. We cannot change the cards we are dealt, just how we play the hand."

In that moment, I was definitely feeling healthy and whole, the Randy of old, powered no doubt by adrenaline and the thrill of a full house. I knew I looked pretty healthy, too, and that some people might have trouble reconciling that with the fact that I was near death. So I addressed it. "If I don't seem as depressed or morose as I should be, sorry to disappoint you," I said, and after people laughed, I added: "I assure you I am not in denial. It's not like I'm not aware of what's going on.

"My family—my three kids, my wife—we just decamped. We bought a lovely house in Virginia, and we're doing that because that's a better place for the family to be down the road." I showed a slide of the new suburban home we'd just purchased. Above the photo of the house was the heading: "I am not in denial."

My point: Jai and I had decided to uproot our family, and I had asked her to leave a home she loved and friends who cared about her. We had taken the kids away from their Pittsburgh playmates. We had packed up our lives, throwing ourselves into a tornado of our own making, when we could have just cocooned in Pittsburgh, waiting for me to die. And we had made this move because we knew that once I was gone, Jai and the kids would need to live in a place where her extended family could help them and love them.

I also wanted the audience to know that I looked good, and felt OK, in part because my body had started to recover from the debilitating chemotherapy and radiation my doctors had been giving me. I was now on the easier-to-endure palliative chemo. "I am in phenomenally good health right now," I said. "I mean, the greatest thing of cognitive dissonance you will ever see is that I am in really good shape. In fact, I am in better shape than most of you."

I moved sideways toward center stage. Hours earlier, I wasn't sure I'd have the strength to do what I was about to do, but now I felt emboldened and potent. I dropped to the floor and began doing push-ups.

In the audience's laughter and surprised applause, it was almost as if I could hear everyone collectively exhaling their anxiety. It wasn't just some dying man. It was just me. I could begin.

II

REALLY ACHIEVING YOUR CHILDHOOD DREAMS

My Childhood Dreams

- Being in zero gravity
- Playing in the NFL
- Authoring an article in the World Book encyclopedia
- Being Captain Kirk
- Winning stuffed animals
- Being a Disney Imagineer

A slide from my talk . . .

4

The Parent Lottery

I WON THE parent lottery.

I was born with the winning ticket, a major reason I was able to live out my childhood dreams.

My mother was a tough, old-school English teacher with nerves of titanium. She worked her students hard, enduring those parents who complained that she expected too much from kids. As her son, I knew a thing or two about her high expectations, and that became my good fortune.

My dad was a World War II medic who served in the Battle of the Bulge. He founded a nonprofit group to help immigrants' kids learn English. And for his livelihood, he ran a small business which sold auto insurance in inner-city Baltimore. His clients were mostly poor people with bad credit histories or few resources, and he'd find a way to get them insured and on the road. For a million reasons, my dad was my hero.

I grew up comfortably middle class in Columbia, Maryland. Money was never an issue in our house, mostly because my parents never saw a need to spend much. They were frugal to a fault. We rarely went out to dinner. We'd see a movie maybe once or twice a year. "Watch TV," my parents would say. "It's free. Or better yet, go to the library. Get a book."

When I was two years old and my sister was four, my mom took us to the circus. I wanted to go again when I was nine. "You don't need to go," my mom said. "You've already been to the circus."

It sounds oppressive by today's standards, but it was actually a magical childhood. I really do see myself as a guy who had this incredible leg up in life because I had a mother and a father who got so many things right.

We didn't buy much. But we thought about everything. That's because my dad had this infectious inquisitiveness about current events, history, our lives. In fact, growing up, I thought there were two types of families:

1) Those who need a dictionary to get through dinner.
2) Those who don't.

We were No. 1. Most every night, we'd end up consulting the dictionary, which we kept on a shelf just six steps from the table. "If you have a question," my folks would say, "then find the answer."

The instinct in our house was never to sit around like slobs and wonder. We knew a better way: Open the encyclopedia. Open the dictionary. Open your mind.

My dad was also an incredible storyteller, and he always

said that stories should be told for a reason. He liked humorous anecdotes that turned into morality tales. He was a master at that kind of story, and I soaked up his techniques. That's why, when my sister, Tammy, watched my last lecture online, she saw my mouth moving, she heard a voice, but it wasn't mine. It was Dad's. She knew I was recycling more than a few of his choicest bits of wisdom. I won't deny that for a second. In fact, at times I felt like I was channeling my dad on stage.

I quote my father to people almost every day. Part of that is because if you dispense your own wisdom, others often dismiss it; if you offer wisdom from a third party, it seems less arrogant and more acceptable. Of course, when you have someone like my dad in your back pocket, you can't help yourself. You quote him every chance you get.

My dad gave me advice on how to negotiate my way through life. He'd say things like: "Never make a decision until you have to." He'd also warn me that even if I was in a position of strength, whether at work or in relationships, I had to play fair. "Just because you're in the driver's seat," he'd say, "doesn't mean you have to run people over."

Lately, I find myself quoting my dad even if it was something he didn't say. Whatever my point, it might as well have come from him. He seemed to know everything.

My mother, meanwhile, knew plenty, too. All my life, she saw it as part of her mission to keep my cockiness in check. I'm grateful for that now. Even these days, if someone asks her what I was like as a kid, she describes me as "alert, but not terribly precocious." We now live in an age when parents praise every child as a genius. And here's my mother, figuring "alert" ought to suffice as a compliment.

When I was studying for my PhD, I took something called "the theory qualifier," which I can now definitively say was the *second* worst thing in my life after chemotherapy. When I complained to my mother about how hard and awful the test was, she leaned over, patted me on the arm and said, "We know just how you feel, honey. And remember, when your father was your age, he was fighting the Germans."

After I got my PhD, my mother took great relish in introducing me by saying: "This is my son. He's a doctor, but not the kind who helps people."

My parents knew what it really took to help people. They were always finding big projects off the beaten path, then throwing themselves into them. Together, they underwrote a fifty-student dormitory in rural Thailand, which was designed to help girls remain in school and avoid prostitution.

My mother was always supremely charitable. And my father would have been happy giving everything away and living in a sack cloth instead of in the suburbs, where the rest of us wanted to live. In that sense, I consider my father the most "Christian" man I've ever met. He was also a huge champion of social equality. Unlike my mom, he didn't easily embrace organized religion. (We were Presbyterians.) He was more focused on the grandest ideals and saw equality as the greatest of goals. He had high hopes for society, and though his hopes were too often dashed, he remained a raging optimist.

At age eighty-three, my dad was diagnosed with leukemia. Knowing he didn't have long to live, he arranged to donate his body to medical science, and he gave money to continue his program in Thailand for at least six more years.

Many people who saw my last lecture were taken with one particular photo that I flashed on the overhead screen: It's a photo in which I'm in my pajamas, leaning on my elbow, and it's so obvious that I was a kid who loved to dream big dreams.

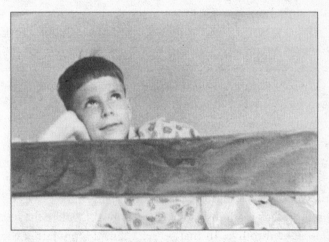

The wood slat that cuts across my body is the front of the bunk bed. My dad, a pretty able woodworker, made me that bed. The smile on that kid's face, the wood slat, the look in his eyes: that photo reminds me that I won the parent lottery.

Although my children will have a loving mother who I know will guide them through life brilliantly, they will not have their father. I've accepted that, but it does hurt.

I'd like to believe my dad would have approved of how I'm going about these last months of my life. He would have advised me to put everything in order for Jai, to spend as much time as possible with the kids—the things I'm doing. I know he would see the sense in moving the family to Virginia.

I also think my dad would be reminding me that kids—more than anything else—need to know their parents love them. Their parents don't have to be alive for that to happen.

5

The Elevator in the Ranch House

M Y IMAGINATION was always pretty hard to contain, and halfway through high school, I felt this urge to splash some of the thoughts swirling in my head onto the walls of my childhood bedroom.

I asked my parents for permission.

"I want to paint things on my walls," I said.

"Like what?" they asked.

"Things that matter to me," I said. "Things I think will be cool. You'll see."

That explanation was enough for my father. That's what was so great about him. He encouraged creativity just by smiling at you. He loved to watch the spark of enthusiasm turn into fireworks. And he understood me and my need to express myself in unconventional ways. So he thought my wall-painting adventure was a great idea.

My mother wasn't so high on the whole escapade, but she relented pretty quickly when she saw how excited I was. She also knew Dad usually won out on these things. She might as well surrender peacefully.

For two days, with the help of my sister, Tammy, and my friend Jack Sheriff, I painted on the walls of my bedroom. My father sat in the living room, reading the newspaper, patiently waiting for the unveiling. My mother hovered in the hallway, completely nervous. She kept sneaking up on us, trying to get a peek, but we remained barricaded in the room. Like they say in the movies, this was "a closed set."

What did we paint?

Well, I wanted to have a quadratic formula on the wall. In a quadratic equation, the highest power of an unknown quantity is a square. Always the nerd, I thought that was worth celebrating. Right by the door, I painted: $\dfrac{-b \pm \sqrt{b^2 - 4ac}}{2a}$

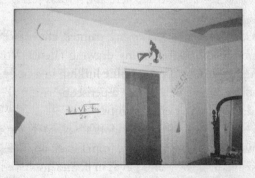

Jack and I painted a large silver elevator door. To the left of the door, we drew "Up" and "Down" buttons, and above the elevator, we painted a panel with floor numbers one through six. The number "three" was illuminated. We lived in a ranch house—it was just one level—so I was doing a bit of fantasizing to imagine six floors. But looking back, why didn't I paint eighty or ninety floors? If I was such a big-shot dreamer, why did my elevator stop at three? I don't know. Maybe it was a symbol of the balance in my life between aspiration and pragmatism.

Given my limited artistic skills, I thought it best if I sketched things out in basic geometric shapes. So I painted a simple rocket ship with fins. I painted Snow White's mirror with the line: "Remember when I told you that you were the fairest? I lied!"

On the ceiling, Jack and I wrote the words "I'm trapped in the attic!" We did the letters backwards, so it seemed as if we'd imprisoned someone up there and he was scratching out an S.O.S.

Because I loved chess, Tammy painted chess pieces (she was the only one of us with any drawing talent). While she handled that, I painted a submarine lurking in a body of water behind the bunk bed. I drew a periscope rising above the bedspread, in search of enemy ships.

I always liked the story of Pandora's box, so Tammy and I painted our version of it. Pandora, from Greek mythology, was given a box with all the world's evils in it. She disobeyed orders not to open it. When the lid came off, evil spread throughout the world. I was always drawn to the story's optimistic ending: Left at the bottom of the box was "hope." So inside my Pandora's box, I wrote the word "Hope." Jack saw that and couldn't resist writing the word "Bob" over "Hope." When friends visited my room, it always took them a minute to figure out why the word "Bob" was there. Then came the inevitable eye-roll.

Given that it was the late 1970s, I wrote the words "Disco sucks!" over my door. My mother thought that was vulgar. One day when I wasn't looking, she quietly painted over the word "sucks." That was the only editing she ever did.

Friends who'd come by were always pretty impressed. "I can't believe your parents let you do this," they'd say.

Though my mother wasn't thrilled at the time, she never painted over the room, even decades after I'd moved out. In fact, over time, my bedroom became the focal point of her house tour when anyone came to visit. My mom began to realize: People thought this was definitely cool. And they thought she was cool for allowing me to do it.

Anybody out there who is a parent, if your kids want to paint their bedrooms, as a favor to me, let them do it. It'll be OK. Don't worry about resale value on the house.

I don't know how many more times I will get to visit my childhood home. But it is a gift every time I go there. I still sleep in that bunk bed my father built, I look at those crazy walls, I think about my parents allowing me to paint, and I fall asleep feeling lucky and pleased.

6

Getting to Zero G

IT'S IMPORTANT to have specific dreams.

When I was in grade school, a lot of kids wanted to become astronauts. I was aware, from an early age, that NASA wouldn't want me. I had heard that astronauts couldn't have glasses. I was OK with that. I didn't really want the whole astronaut gig. I just wanted the floating.

Turns out that NASA has a plane it uses to help astronauts acclimate to zero gravity. Everyone calls it "the Vomit Comet," even though NASA refers to it as "The Weightless Wonder," a public-relations gesture aimed at distracting attention from the obvious.

Whatever the plane is called, it's a sensational piece of machinery. It does parabolic arcs, and at the top of each arc, you get about twenty-five seconds when you experience the rough equivalent of weightlessness. As the plane dives, you feel like you're on a runaway roller coaster, but you're suspended, flying around.

My dream became a possibility when I learned that NASA had a program in which college students could submit proposals for experiments on the plane. In 2001, our team of Carnegie Mellon students proposed a project using virtual reality.

Being weightless is a sensation hard to fathom when you've been an Earthling all your life. In zero gravity, the inner ear, which controls balance, isn't quite in synch with what your eyes are telling you. Nausea is often the result. Could virtual reality dry-runs on the ground help? That was the question in our proposal, and it was a winner. We were invited to Johnson Space Center in Houston to ride the plane.

I was probably more excited than any of my students. Floating! But late in the process, I got bad news. NASA made it very clear that under no circumstances could faculty advisors fly with their students.

I was heartbroken, but I was not deterred. I would find a way around this brick wall. I decided to carefully read all the literature about the program, looking for loopholes. And I found one: NASA, always eager for good publicity, would allow a journalist from the students' hometown to come along for the ride.

I called an official at NASA to ask for his fax number. "What are you going to fax us?" he asked. I explained: my resignation as the faculty advisor and my application as the journalist.

"I'll be accompanying my students in my new role as a member of the media," I said.

And he said, "That's a little transparent, don't you think?"

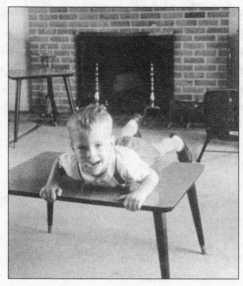

I just wanted the floating . . .

"Sure," I said, but I also promised him that I'd get information about our experiment onto news Web sites, and send film of our virtual reality efforts to more mainstream journalists. I knew I could pull that off, and it was win-win for everyone. He gave me his fax number.

As an aside, there's a lesson here: Have something to bring to the table, because that will make you more welcome.

My experience in zero G was spectacular (and no, I didn't throw up, thank you). I did get banged up a bit, though, because at the end of the magical twenty-five seconds, when gravity returns to the plane, it's actually as if you've become twice your weight. You can slam down pretty hard. That's why we were repeatedly told: "Feet down!" You don't want to crash land on your neck.

But I did manage to get on that plane, almost four decades after floating became one of my life goals. It just proves that if you can find an opening, you can probably find a way to float through it.

7

I Never Made It to the NFL

I LOVE FOOTBALL. *Tackle* football. I started playing when I was nine years old, and football got me through. It helped make me who I am today. And even though I did not reach the National Football League, I sometimes think I got more from pursuing that dream, and *not* accomplishing it, then I did from many of the ones I did accomplish.

My romance with football started when my dad dragged me, kicking and screaming, to join a league. I had no desire to be there. I was naturally wimpy, and the smallest kid by far. Fear turned to awe when I met my coach, Jim Graham, a hulking, six-foot-four wall-of-a-guy. He had been a linebacker at Penn State, and was seriously old-school. I mean, *really* old-school; like he thought the forward pass was a trick play.

On the first day of practice, we were all scared to death. Plus he hadn't brought along any footballs. One kid finally spoke up for all of us. "Excuse me, Coach. There are no footballs."

And Coach Graham responded, "We don't need any foot-balls."

There was a silence, while we thought about that . . .

"How many men are on the football field at a time?" he asked us.

Eleven on a team, we answered. So that makes twenty-two.

"And how many people are touching the football at any given time?"

One of them.

"Right!" he said. "So we're going to work on what those *other* twenty-one guys are doing."

Fundamentals. That was a great gift Coach Graham gave us. Fundamentals, fundamentals, fundamentals. As a college professor, I've seen this as one lesson so many kids ignore, always to their detriment: You've *got* to get the fundamentals down, because otherwise the fancy stuff is not going to work.

* * *

Coach Graham used to ride me hard. I remember one prac-tice in particular. "You're doing it all wrong, Pausch. Go back! Do it again!" I tried to do what he wanted. It wasn't enough. "You owe me, Pausch! You're doing push-ups after practice."

When I was finally dismissed, one of the assistant coaches came over to reassure me. "Coach Graham rode you pretty hard, didn't he?" he said.

I could barely muster a "yeah."

"That's a good thing," the assistant told me. "When

you're screwing up and nobody says anything to you anymore, that means they've given up on you."

That lesson has stuck with me my whole life. When you see yourself doing something badly and nobody's bothering to tell you anymore, that's a bad place to be. You may not want to hear it, but your critics are often the ones telling you they still love you and care about you, and want to make you better.

There's a lot of talk these days about giving children self-esteem. It's not something you can *give;* it's something they have to build. Coach Graham worked in a no-coddling zone. Self-esteem? He knew there was really only one way to teach kids how to develop it: You give them something they can't do, they work hard until they find they can do it, and you just keep repeating the process.

When Coach Graham first got hold of me, I was this wimpy kid with no skills, no physical strength, and no conditioning. But he made me realize that if I work hard enough, there will be things I can do tomorrow that I can't do today. Even now, having just turned forty-seven, I can give you a three-point stance that any NFL lineman would be proud of.

I realize that, these days, a guy like Coach Graham might get thrown out of a youth sports league. He'd be too tough. Parents would complain.

I remember one game when our team was playing terribly. At halftime, in our rush for water, we almost knocked over the water bucket. Coach Graham was livid: "Jeez! That's the most I've seen you boys move since this game started!" We were eleven years old, just standing there, afraid he'd pick us up one by one and break us with his bare hands. "Water?" he barked. "You boys want water?" He lifted the bucket and dumped all the water on the ground.

We watched him walk away and heard him mutter to an assistant coach: "You can give water to the first-string defense. They played OK."

Now let me be clear: Coach Graham would never endanger any kid. One reason he worked so hard on conditioning was he knew it reduces injuries. However, it was a chilly day, we'd all had access to water during the first half, and the dash to the water bucket was more about us being a bunch of brats than really needing hydration.

Even so, if that kind of incident happened today, parents on the sidelines would be pulling out their cell phones to call the league commissioner, or maybe their lawyer.

It saddens me that many kids today are so coddled. I think back to how I felt during that halftime rant. Yes, I was thirsty. But more than that, I felt humiliated. We had all let down Coach Graham, and he let us know it in a way we'd never forget. He was right. We had shown more energy at the water bucket than we had in the damn game. And getting chewed out by him meant something to us. During the second half, we went back on the field, and gave it our all.

I haven't seen Coach Graham since I was a teen, but he just keeps showing up in my head, forcing me to work harder whenever I feel like quitting, forcing me to be better. He gave me a feedback loop for life.

* * *

When we send our kids to play organized sports—football, soccer, swimming, whatever—for most of us, it's not because we're desperate for them to learn the intricacies of the sport.

What we really want them to learn is far more important: teamwork, perseverance, sportsmanship, the value of hard work, an ability to deal with adversity. This kind of indirect learning is what some of us like to call a "head fake."

There are two kinds of head fakes. The first is literal. On a football field, a player will move his head one way so you'll think he's going in that direction. Then he goes the opposite way. It's like a magician using misdirection. Coach Graham used to tell us to watch a player's waist. "Where his belly button goes, his body goes," he'd say.

The second kind of head fake is the *really* important one—the one that teaches people things they don't realize they're learning until well into the process. If you're a head-fake specialist, your hidden objective is to get them to learn something you want them to learn.

This kind of head-fake learning is absolutely vital. And Coach Graham was the master.

8

You'll Find Me Under "V"

I LIVE IN the computer age and I love it here! I have long embraced pixels, multi-screen work stations and the information superhighway. I really can picture a paperless world.

And yet, I grew up in a very different place.

When I was born in 1960, paper was where great knowledge was recorded. In my house, all through the 1960s and 1970s, our family worshipped the World Book Encyclopedia—the photos, the maps, the flags of different countries, the handy sidebars revealing each state's population, motto and average elevation.

I didn't read every word of every volume of the World Book, but I gave it a shot. I was fascinated by how it all came together. Who wrote that section on the aardvark? How that must have been, to have the World Book editors call and say, "You know aardvarks better than anyone. Would you write an entry for us?" Then there was the Z volume. Who was the person deemed enough of a Zulu expert to create that entry? Was he or she a Zulu?

My parents were frugal. Unlike many Americans, they would never buy anything for the purposes of impressing other people, or as any kind of luxury for themselves. But they happily bought the World Book, spending a princely sum at the time, because by doing so, they were giving the gift of knowledge to me and my sister. They also ordered the annual companion volumes. Each year, a new volume of break-throughs and current events would arrive—labeled 1970, 1971, 1972, 1973—and I couldn't wait to read them. These annual volumes came with stickers, referencing entries in the original, alphabetical World Books. My job was to attach those stickers on the appropriate pages, and I took that responsibility seriously. I was helping to chronicle history and science for anyone who opened those encyclopedias in the future.

Given how I cherished the World Book, one of my childhood dreams was to be a contributor. But it's not like you can call World Book headquarters in Chicago and suggest yourself. The World Book has to find you.

A few years ago, believe it or not, the call finally came.

It turned out that somehow, my career up to that time had turned me into exactly the sort of expert that World Book felt comfortable badgering. They didn't think I was the most important virtual reality expert in the world. That person was too busy for them to approach. But me, I was in that midrange level—just respectable enough . . . but not so famous that I'd turn them down.

"Would you like to write our new entry on virtual reality?" they asked.

I couldn't tell them that I'd been waiting all my life for this call. All I could say was, "Yes, of course!" I wrote the entry. And I included a photo of my student Caitlin Kelleher wearing a virtual reality headset.

No editor ever questioned what I wrote, but I assume that's the World Book way. They pick an expert and trust that the expert won't abuse the privilege.

I have not bought the latest set of World Books. In fact, having been selected to be an author in the World Book, I now believe that Wikipedia is a perfectly fine source for your information, because I know what the quality control is for real encyclopedias. But sometimes when I'm in a library with the kids, I still can't resist looking under "V" ("Virtual Reality" by yours truly) and letting them have a look. Their dad made it.

9

A Skill Set Called Leadership

LIKE COUNTLESS American nerds born in 1960, I spent part of my childhood dreaming of being Captain James T. Kirk, commander of the Starship *Enterprise*. I didn't see myself as Captain Pausch. I imagined a world where I actually got to *be* Captain Kirk.

For ambitious young boys with a scientific bent, there could be no greater role model than James T. Kirk of *Star Trek*. In fact, I seriously believe that I became a better teacher and colleague—maybe even a better husband—by watching Kirk run the *Enterprise*.

Think about it. If you've seen the TV show, you know that Kirk was not the smartest guy on the ship. Mr. Spock, his first officer, was the always-logical intellect on board. Dr. McCoy had all the medical knowledge available to mankind in the 2260s. Scotty was the chief engineer, who had the technical know-how to keep that ship running, even when it was under attack by aliens.

So what was Kirk's skill set? Why did he get to climb on board the *Enterprise* and run it?

The answer: There is this skill set called "leadership."

I learned so much by watching this guy in action. He was the distilled essence of the dynamic manager, a guy who knew how to delegate, had the passion to inspire, and looked good in what he wore to work. He never professed to have skills greater than his subordinates. He acknowledged that they knew what they were doing in their domains. But he established the vision, the tone. He was in charge of morale. On top of that, Kirk had the romantic chops to woo women in every galaxy he visited. Picture me at home watching TV, a ten-year-old in glasses. Every time Kirk showed up on the screen he was like a Greek god to me.

And he had the coolest damn toys! When I was a kid, I thought it was fascinating that he could be on some planet and he had this thing—this Star Trek communicator device—that let him talk to people back on the ship. I now walk around with one in my pocket. Who remembers that it was Kirk who introduced us to the cell phone?

A few years ago, I got a call (on my communicator device) from a Pittsburgh author named Chip Walter. He was co-writing a book with William Shatner (a.k.a. Kirk) about how scientific breakthroughs first imagined on *Star Trek* foreshadowed today's technological advancements. Captain Kirk wanted to visit my virtual reality lab at Carnegie Mellon.

Granted, my childhood dream was to *be* Kirk. But I still

considered it a dream realized when Shatner showed up. It's cool to meet your boyhood idol, but it's almost indescribably cooler when he comes to you to see cool stuff you're doing in your lab.

My students and I worked around the clock to build a virtual reality world that resembled the bridge of the Enterprise. When Shatner arrived, we put this bulky "head-mounted display" on him. It had a screen inside, and as he turned his head, he could immerse himself in 360-degree images of his old ship. "Wow, you even have the turbolift doors," he said. And we had a surprise for him, too: red-alert sirens. Without missing a beat, he barked, "We're under attack!"

Shatner stayed for three hours and asked tons of questions. A colleague later said to me: "He just kept asking and asking. He doesn't seem to get it."

But I was hugely impressed. Kirk, I mean, Shatner, was the ultimate example of a man who knew what he didn't know, was perfectly willing to admit it, and didn't want to leave until he understood. That's heroic to me. I wish every grad student had that attitude.

During my cancer treatment, when I was told that only 4 percent of pancreatic cancer patients live five years, a line from the Star Trek movie *The Wrath of Khan* came into my head. In the film, Starfleet cadets are faced with a simulated training scenario where, no matter what they do, their entire crew is killed. The film explains that when Kirk was a cadet, he reprogrammed the simulation because "he didn't believe in the no-win scenario."

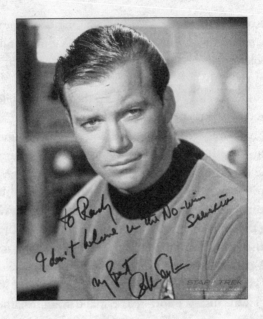

Over the years, some of my sophisticated academic colleagues have turned up their noses at my Star Trek infatuation. But from the start, it has never failed to stand me in good stead.

After Shatner learned of my diagnosis, he sent me a photo of himself as Kirk. On it he wrote: "I don't believe in the no-win scenario."

10

Winning Big

ONE OF my earliest childhood dreams was to be the coolest guy at any amusement park or carnival I visited. I always knew exactly how that kind of coolness was achieved.

The coolest guy was easy to spot: He was the one walking around with the largest stuffed animal. As a kid, I'd see some guy off in the distance with his head and body mostly hidden by an enormous stuffed animal. It didn't matter if he was a buffed-up Adonis, or if he was some nerd who couldn't get his arms around it. If he had the biggest stuffed animal, then he was the coolest guy at the carnival.

My dad subscribed to the same belief. He felt naked on a Ferris wheel if he didn't have a huge, newly won bear or ape on his hip. Given the competitiveness in our family, midway games became a battle. Which one of us could capture the largest beast in the Stuffed Animal Kingdom?

Have you ever walked around a carnival with a giant stuffed animal? Have you ever watched how people look at you and envy you? Have you ever used a stuffed animal to woo a woman? I have . . . and I married her!

Giant stuffed animals have played a role in my life from the start. There was that time when I was three years old and my sister was five. We were in a store's toy department, and my father said he'd buy us any one item if we could agree on it and share it. We looked around and around, and eventually we looked up and saw, on the highest shelf, a giant stuffed rabbit.

"We'll take that!" my sister said.

It was probably the most expensive item in the toy department. But my father was a man of his word. And so he bought it for us. He likely figured it was a good investment. A home could always use another giant stuffed animal.

As I reached adulthood and kept showing up with more and bigger stuffed animals, my father suspected that I was paying people off. He assumed that I was waiting for winners over by the squirt guns, and then slipping a fifty to some guy who didn't realize how a giant stuffed animal could change the world's perception of him. But I never paid for a stuffed animal.

And I never cheated.

OK, I admit that I leaned. That's the only way to do it at the ring toss. I am a leaner, but I am not a cheater.

I did, however, do a lot of my winning out of view of my family. And I know that increased suspicions. But I found the best way to bag stuffed animals is without the pressure of a family audience. I also didn't want anyone to know just how long it took me to be successful. Tenacity is a virtue, but it's not always crucial for everyone to observe how hard you work at something.

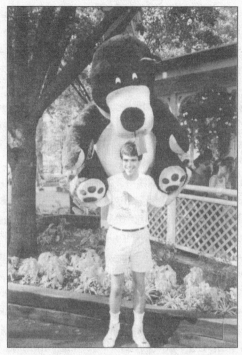

Have you ever walked around a carnival with a
giant stuffed animal?

I am prepared now to reveal that there are two secrets to
winning giant stuffed animals: long arms and a small amount of
discretionary income. I have been blessed in life to have both.

I talked about my stuffed animals at my last lecture, and
showed photos of them. I could predict what the tech-savvy

cynics were thinking: In this age of digitally manipulated images, maybe those stuffed bears weren't really in the pictures
with me. Or maybe I sweet-talked the actual winners into letting me have my photo taken next to their prizes.

How, in this age of cynicism, could I convince my audience that I'd really won these things? Well, I would show
them the actual stuffed animals. And so I had some of my
students walk in from the wings of the stage, each carrying a
giant stuffed animal I'd won over the years.

I don't need these trophies anymore. And although I
know my wife loved the stuffed bear I'd hung in her office
when we were courting, three children later, she doesn't want
an army of them cluttering up our new house. (They were
leaking styrofoam beads that were making their way into
Chloe's mouth.)

I knew that if I kept the stuffed animals, someday Jai
would be calling Goodwill and saying, "Take them away!" . . .
or worse, feeling she couldn't! That's why I had decided: Why
don't I give them to friends?

And so once they were lined up on stage, I announced:
"Anybody who would like a piece of me at the end of this,
feel free to come up and take a bear; first come, first served."

The giant stuffed animals all found homes quickly. A few
days later, I learned that one of the animals had been taken
by a Carnegie Mellon student who, like me, has cancer. After
the lecture, she walked up and selected the giant elephant. I
love the symbolism of that. She got the elephant in the room.

II

The Happiest Place on Earth

IN 1969, when I was eight years old, my family went on a cross-country trip to see Disneyland. It was an absolute quest. And once we got there, I was just in awe of the place. It was the coolest environment I'd ever been in.

As I stood in line with all the other kids, all I could think was "I can't wait to make stuff like this!"

Two decades later, when I got my PhD in computer science from Carnegie Mellon, I thought that made me infinitely qualified to do anything, so I dashed off my letters of application to Walt Disney Imagineering. And they sent me some of the *nicest* go-to-hell letters I'd ever received. They said they had reviewed my application, and they did not have "any positions which require your particular qualifications."

Nothing? This is a company famous for hiring armies of people to sweep the streets! Disney had nothing for me? Not even a broom?

So that was a setback. But I kept my mantra in mind: The brick walls are there for a reason. They're not there to keep us out. The brick walls are there to give us a chance to show how badly we want something.

Fast-forward to 1995. I'd become a professor at the University of Virginia, and I'd helped build a system called "Virtual Reality on Five Dollars a Day." This was at a time when virtual reality experts were insisting they'd need a half-million dollars to do anything. And my colleagues and I did our own little version of the Hewlett-Packard garage thing and hacked together a working low-budget virtual reality system. People in the computer science world thought this was pretty great.

Not too long after, I learned that Disney Imagineering was working on a virtual reality project. It was top secret, and it was an Aladdin attraction that would allow people to ride a magic carpet. I called Disney and explained that I was a virtual reality researcher looking for information on it. I was ridiculously persistent, and I kept getting passed on and on until I was connected to a guy named Jon Snoddy. He happened to be the brilliant Imagineer running the team. I felt as if I had called the White House and been put through to the president.

After we chatted a while, I told Jon I'd be coming to California. Could we get together? (Truth was, if he said yes, the only reason I'd be coming would be to see him. I'd have gone to *Neptune* to see him!) He told me OK. If I was coming anyway, we could have lunch.

Before going to see him, I did eighty hours of homework. I asked all the virtual reality hotshots I knew to share their thoughts and questions about this Disney project. As a result, when I finally met Jon, he was wowed by how prepared I was. (It's easy to look smart when you're parroting smart people.) Then, at the end of the lunch, I made "the ask."

"I have a sabbatical coming up," I said.

"What's that?" he asked, which was my first hint of the academic/entertainment culture clash I'd be facing.

After I explained the concept of sabbaticals, he thought it would be a fine idea to have me spend mine with his team. The deal was: I'd come for six months, work on a project, and publish a paper about it. I was thrilled. It was almost unheard of for Imagineering to invite an academic like me inside their secretive operation.

The only problem: I needed permission from my bosses to take this kind of oddball sabbatical.

Well, every Disney story needs a villain, and mine happened to be a certain dean from the University of Virginia. "Dean Wormer" (as Jai dubbed him in homage to the film *Animal House*) was concerned that Disney would suck all this "intellectual property" out of my head that rightfully belonged to the university. He argued against my doing it. I asked him: "Do you think this is a good idea at all?" And he said: "I have no idea if it is a good idea." He was proof that, sometimes, the most impenetrable brick walls are made of flesh.

Because I was getting nowhere with him, I took my case to the dean of sponsored research. I asked him: "Do you think it's a good idea that I do this?" And he answered: "I don't have enough information to say. But I do know that one of my star

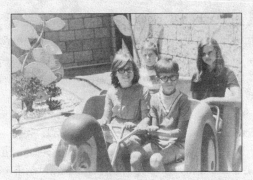

My sister and me on the Alice ride: All I could
think was, "I can't wait to make stuff like this."

faculty members is in my office and he's really excited. So tell
me more."

Now, here's a lesson for managers and administrators.
Both deans said the same thing: They didn't know if this sabbatical was a good idea. But think about how differently they
said it!

I ended up being allowed to take that sabbatical, and it
was a fantasy come true. In fact, I have a confession. This is
exactly how geeky I am: Soon after I arrived in California, I
hopped into my convertible and drove over to Imagineering
headquarters. It was a hot summer night, and I had the
soundtrack to Disney's *The Lion King* blasting on my stereo.
Tears actually began streaming down my face as I drove past
the building. Here I was, the grown-up version of that wide-
eyed eight-year-old at Disneyland. I had finally arrived. I was
an Imagineer.

III

ADVENTURES ...
AND LESSONS
LEARNED

12

The Park Is Open *Until 8 p.m.*

My medical odyssey began in the summer of 2006, when I first felt slight, unexplained pain in my upper abdomen. Later, jaundice set in, and my doctors suspected I had hepatitis. That turned out to be wishful thinking. CT scans revealed I had pancreatic cancer, and it would take me just ten seconds on Google to discover how bad this news was. Pancreatic cancer has the highest mortality rate of any cancer; half of those diagnosed with it die within six months, and 96 percent die within five years.

I approached my treatment like I approach so many things, as a scientist. And so I asked lots of data-seeking questions, and found myself hypothesizing along with my doctors. I made audio tapes of my conversations with them, so I could listen more closely to their explanations at home. I'd find obscure journal articles and bring them with me to appointments. Doctors didn't seem to be put off by me. In fact, most thought I was a fun patient because I was so engaged in everything. (They even didn't seem to mind when I brought along advocates—my friend and colleague Jessica Hodgins came to appointments to offer both support and her brilliant research skills in navigating medical information.)

I told doctors that I'd be willing to endure anything in their surgical arsenal, and I'd swallow anything in their medicine cabinet, because I had an objective: I wanted to be alive as long as possible for Jai and the kids. At my first appointment with Pittsburgh surgeon Herb Zeh, I said: "Let's be clear. My goal is to be alive and on your brochure in ten years."

I turned out to be among the minority of patients who could benefit from what is called the "Whipple operation," named for a doctor who in the 1930s conjured up this complicated procedure. Through the 1970s, the surgery itself was killing up to 25 percent of patients who underwent it. By the year 2000, the risk of dying from it was under 5 percent if done by experienced specialists. Still, I knew I was in for a brutal time, especially since the surgery needed to be followed by an extremely toxic regimen of chemotherapy and radiation.

As part of the surgery, Dr. Zeh removed not only the tumor, but my gallbladder, a third of my pancreas, a third of my stomach, and several feet of my small intestine. Once I recovered from that, I spent two months at MD Anderson Cancer Center in Houston, receiving those powerful dosages of chemo, plus daily high-dose radiation of my abdomen. I went from 182 to 138 pounds and, by the end, could hardly walk. In January, I went home to Pittsburgh and my CT scans showed no cancer. I slowly regained my strength.

In August, it was time for my quarterly check-in back at

MD Anderson. Jai and I flew to Houston for the appointment, leaving the kids with a babysitter back home. We treated the trip like something of a romantic getaway. We even went to a giant water park the day before—I know, my idea of a romantic getaway—and I rode the speed slide, grinning all the way down.

Then, on August 15, 2007, a Wednesday, Jai and I arrived at MD Anderson to go over the results of my latest CT scans with my oncologist, Robert Wolff. We were ushered into an examining room, where a nurse asked a few routine questions. "Any changes in your weight, Randy? Are you still taking the same medications?" Jai took note of the nurse's happy, singsong voice as she left, how she cheerily said, "OK, the doctor will be in to see you soon," as she closed the door behind her.

The examining room had a computer in it, and I noticed that the nurse hadn't logged out; my medical records were still up on the screen. I know my way around computers, of course, but this required no hacking at all. My whole chart was right there.

"Shall we have a look-see?" I said to Jai. I felt no qualms at all about what I was about to do. After all, these were my records.

I clicked around and found my blood-work report. There were 30 obscure blood values, but I knew the one I was looking for: CA 19-9—the tumor marker. When I found it, the number was a horrifying 208. A normal value is under 37. I studied it for just a second.

"It's over," I said to Jai. "My goose is cooked."

"What do you mean?" she asked.

I told her the CA 19-9 value. She had educated herself enough about cancer treatment to know that 208 indicated metastasis: a death sentence. "It's not funny," she said. "Stop joking around."

I then pulled up my CT scans on the computer and started counting. "One, two, three, four, five, six . . ."

I could hear the panic in Jai's voice. "Don't tell me you're counting tumors," she said. I couldn't help myself. I kept counting aloud. "Seven, eight, nine, ten . . ." I saw it all. The cancer had metastasized to my liver.

Jai walked over to the computer, saw everything clearly with her own eyes, and fell into my arms. We cried together. And that's when I realized there was no box of tissues in the room. I had just learned I would soon die, and in my inability to stop being rationally focused, I found myself thinking: "Shouldn't a room like this, at a time like this, have a box of Kleenex? Wow, that's a glaring operational flaw."

There was a knock on the door. Dr. Wolff entered, a folder in his hand. He looked from Jai to me to the CT scans on the computer, and he knew what had just happened. I decided to just be preemptive. "We know," I said.

By that point, Jai was almost in shock, crying hysterically. I was sad, too, of course, and yet I was also fascinated by the way in which Dr. Wolff went about the grim task before him. The doctor sat next to Jai to comfort her. Calmly, he explained to her that he would no longer be working to save my life. "What we're trying to do," he said, "is extend the time Randy has left so he can have the highest quality of life. That's because, as things now stand, medical science doesn't have anything to offer him to keep him alive for a normal life span."

"Wait, wait, wait," Jai said. "You're telling me that's it? Just like that, we've gone from 'we're going to fight this' to 'the battle is over'? What about a liver transplant?"

No, the doctor said, not once the metastasis occurs. He talked about using palliative chemo—treatment that's not intended to be curative, but could ease symptoms, possibly buying a few months—and about finding ways to keep me comfortable and engaged in life as the end approached.

The whole horrible exchange was surreal for me. Yes, I felt stunned and bereft for myself and especially for Jai, who couldn't stop crying. But a strong part of me remained in Randy Scientist Mode, collecting facts and quizzing the doctor about options. At the same time, there was another part of me that was utterly engaged in the theater of the moment. I felt incredibly impressed—awed really—by the way Dr. Wolff was giving the news to Jai. I thought to myself: "Look at how he's doing this. He's obviously done this so many times before, and he's good at it. He's carefully rehearsed, and yet everything is still so heartfelt and spontaneous."

I took note of how the doctor rocked back in his chair and closed his eyes before answering a question, almost as if that was helping him think harder. I watched the doctor's body posture, the way he sat next to Jai. I found myself almost detached from it all, thinking: "He isn't putting his arm around her shoulder. I understand why. That would be too presumptuous. But he's leaning in, his hand on her knee. Boy, he's good at this."

I wished every medical student considering oncology could see what I was seeing. I watched Dr. Wolff use semantics to phrase whatever he could in a positive light. When we asked, "How long before I die?" he answered, "You probably have three to six months of good health." That reminded me of my time at Disney. Ask Disney World workers: "What time does the park close?" They're supposed to answer: "The park is *open* until 8 p.m."

In a way, I felt an odd sense of relief. For too many tense months, Jai and I had been waiting to see if and when the tumors would return. Now here they were, a full army of them. The wait was over. Now we could move on to dealing with whatever came next.

At the end of the meeting, the doctor hugged Jai and shook my hand, and Jai and I walked out together, into our new reality.

Leaving the doctor's office, I thought about what I'd said to Jai in the water park in the afterglow of the speed slide. "Even if the scan results are bad tomorrow," I had told her, "I just want you to know that it feels great to be alive, and to be here today, alive with you. Whatever news we get about the scans, I'm not going to die when we hear it. I won't die the next day, or the day after that, or the day after that. So today, right now, well this is a wonderful day. And I want you to know how much I'm enjoying it."

I thought about that, and about Jai's smile.

I knew then. That's the way the rest of my life would need to be lived.

13

The Man in the Convertible

***

ONE MORNING, well after I was diagnosed with cancer, I got an email from Robbee Kosak, Carnegie Mellon's vice president for advancement. She told me a story.

She said she had been driving home from work the night before, and she found herself behind a man in a convertible. It was a warm, gorgeous, early-spring evening, and the man had his top down and all his windows lowered. His arm was hanging over the driver's side door, and his fingers were tapping along to the music on his radio. His head was bobbing along, too, as the wind blew through his hair.

Robbee changed lanes and pulled a little closer. From the side, she could see that the man had a slight smile on his face, the kind of absentminded smile a person might have when he's all alone, happy in his own thoughts. Robbee found herself thinking: "Wow, this is the epitome of a person appreciating this day and this moment."

The convertible eventually turned the corner, and that's

when Robbee got a look at the man's full face. "Oh my God," she said to herself. "It's Randy Pausch!"

She was so struck by the sight of me. She knew that my cancer diagnosis was grim. And yet, as she wrote in her email, she was moved by how contented I seemed. In this private moment, I was obviously in high spirits. Robbee wrote in her email: "You can never know how much that glimpse of you made my day, reminding me of what life is all about."

I read Robbee's email several times. I came to look at it as a feedback loop of sorts.

It has not always been easy to stay positive through my cancer treatment. When you have a dire medical issue, it's tough to know how you're really faring emotionally. I had wondered whether a part of me was acting when I was with other people. Maybe at times I forced myself to appear strong and upbeat. Many cancer patients feel obliged to put up a brave front. Was I doing that, too?

But Robbee had come upon me in an unguarded moment. I'd like to think she saw me as I am. She certainly saw me as I was that evening.

Her email was just a paragraph, but it meant a great deal to me. She had given me a window into myself. I was still fully engaged. I still knew life was good. I was doing OK.

14

The Dutch Uncle

Anyone who knows me will tell you I've always had a healthy sense of myself and my abilities. I tend to say what I'm thinking and what I believe. I don't have much patience for incompetence.

These are traits that have mostly served me well. But there are times, believe it or not, when I've come across as arrogant and tactless. That's when those who can help you recalibrate yourself become absolutely crucial.

My sister, Tammy, had to put up with the ultimate know-it-all kid brother. I was always telling her what to do, as if our birth order was a mistake that I was incessantly trying to correct.

One time when I was seven years old and Tammy was nine, we were waiting for the school bus, and as usual, I was mouthing off. She decided she'd had enough. She picked up my metal lunch box and dropped it in a mud puddle . . . just as the bus pulled up. My sister ended up in the principal's office, while I was sent to the janitor, who cleaned up my lunch box, threw out my mud-soaked sandwich and kindly gave me lunch money.

The principal told Tammy he had called our mother. "I'm going to let her handle this," he said. When we arrived home after school, Mom said, "I'm going to let your father handle this." My sister spent the day nervously awaiting her fate.

When my father got home after work, he listened to the story and burst into a smile. He wasn't going to punish Tammy. He did everything but congratulate her! I was a kid who *needed* to have his lunch box dropped in a puddle. Tammy was relieved, and I'd been put in my place . . . though the lesson didn't completely sink in.

By the time I got to Brown University, I had certain abilities and people knew I knew it. My good friend Scott Sherman, whom I met freshman year, now recalls me as "having a total lack of tact, and being universally acclaimed as the person quickest to offend someone he had just met."

I usually didn't notice how I was coming off, in part because things seemed to be working out and I was succeeding academically. Andy van Dam, the school's legendary computer science professor, made me his teaching assistant. "Andy van Demand," as he was known, liked me. I was impassioned about so many things—a good trait. But like many people, I had strengths that were also flaws. In Andy's view, I was self-possessed to a fault, I was way too brash and I was an inflexible contrarian, always spouting opinions.

One day Andy took me for a walk. He put his arm around my shoulders and said, "Randy, it's such a shame that people perceive you as being so arrogant, because it's going to limit what you're going to be able to accomplish in life."

Looking back, his wording was so perfect. He was actually saying, "Randy, you're being a jerk." But he said it in a way that made me open to his criticisms, to listening to my hero telling me something I needed to hear. There is an old expression, "a Dutch uncle," which refers to a person who gives you honest feedback. Few people bother doing that nowadays, so the expression has started to feel outdated, even obscure. (And the best part is that Andy really *is* Dutch.)

Ever since my last lecture began spreading on the Internet, more than a few friends have been ribbing me about it, calling me "St. Randy." It's their way of reminding me that there were times I've been described in other, more colorful, ways.

But I like to think that my flaws are in the social, rather than in the moral category. And I've been lucky enough to benefit over the years from people like Andy, who have cared enough to tell me the tough-love things that I needed to hear.

15

Pouring Soda in the Backseat

FOR A long time, a big part of my identity was "bachelor uncle." In my twenties and thirties I had no kids, and my sister's two children, Chris and Laura, became the objects of my affection. I reveled in being Uncle Randy, the guy who showed up in their lives every month or so to help them look at their world from strange new angles.

It wasn't that I spoiled them. I just tried to impart my perspective on life. Sometimes that drove my sister crazy.

Once, about a dozen years ago, when Chris was seven years old and Laura was nine, I picked them up in my brand-new Volkswagen Cabrio convertible. "Be careful in Uncle Randy's new car," my sister told them. "Wipe your feet before you get in it. Don't mess anything up. Don't get it dirty."

I listened to her, and thought, as only a bachelor uncle can: "That's just the sort of admonition that sets kids up for failure. Of course they'd eventually get my car dirty. Kids can't help it." So I made things easy. While my sister was outlining the rules, I slowly and deliberately opened a can of soda, turned it over, and poured it on the cloth seats in the back of the convertible. My message: People are more important than things. A car, even a pristine gem like my new convertible, was just a thing.

As I poured out that Coke, I watched Chris and Laura, mouths open, eyes widening. Here was crazy Uncle Randy completely rejecting adult rules.

I ended up being so glad I'd spilled that soda. Because later in the weekend, little Chris got the flu and threw up all over the backseat. He didn't feel guilty. He was relieved; he had already watched *me* christen the car. He knew it would be OK.

Whenever the kids were with me, we had just two rules:

1) No whining.
2) Whatever we do together, don't tell Mom.

Not telling Mom made everything we did into a pirate adventure. Even the mundane could feel magical.

On most weekends, Chris and Laura would hang out at my apartment and I'd take them to Chuck E. Cheese, or we'd head out for a hike or visit a museum. On special weekends, we'd stay in a hotel with a pool.

The three of us liked making pancakes together. My father had always asked: "Why do pancakes need to be round?" I'd ask the same question. And so we were always making weirdly shaped animal pancakes. There's a sloppiness to that medium that I like, because every animal pancake you make is an unintentional Rorschach test. Chris and Laura would say, "This isn't the shape of the animal I wanted." But that allowed us to look at the pancake as it was, and imagine what animal it might be.

I've watched Laura and Chris grow into terrific young adults. She's now twenty-one and he's nineteen. These days, I am more grateful than ever that I was a part of their childhoods, because I've come to realize something. It's unlikely that I will ever get to be a father to children over age six. So my time with Chris and Laura has become even more precious. They gave me the gift of being a presence in their lives through their pre-teen and teen years, and into adulthood.

Recently, I asked both Chris and Laura to do me a favor. After I die, I want them to take my kids for weekends here and there, and just do stuff. Anything fun they can think of. They don't have to do the exact things we did together. They can let my kids take the lead. Dylan likes dinosaurs. Maybe Chris and Laura can take him to a natural history museum. Logan likes sports: maybe they can take him to see the Steelers. And Chloe loves to dance. They'll figure something out.

I also want my niece and nephew to tell my kids a few things. First, they can say simply: "Your dad asked us to spend this time with you, just like he spent time with us." I hope they'll also explain to my kids how hard I fought to stay alive. I signed up for the hardest treatments that could be thrown at me because I wanted to be around as long as possible to be there for my kids. That's the message I've asked Laura and Chris to deliver.

Oh, and one more thing. If my kids mess up their cars, I hope Chris and Laura will think of me and smile.

16

Romancing the Brick Wall

———————

THE MOST formidable brick wall I ever came upon in my life was just five feet, six inches tall, and was absolutely beautiful. But it reduced me to tears, made me reevaluate my entire life and led me to call my father, in a helpless fit, to ask for guidance on how to scale it.

That brick wall was Jai.

As I said in the lecture, I was always pretty adept at charging through the brick walls in my academic and professional life. I didn't tell the audience the story about my courtship with my wife because I knew I'd get too emotional. Still, the words I said on stage completely applied to my early days with Jai:

". . . The brick walls are there to stop the people who don't want it badly enough. They're there to stop the *other* people."

I was a thirty-seven-year-old bachelor when Jai and I met. I'd spent a lot of time dating around, having great fun, and then losing girlfriends who wanted to get more serious. For years, I felt no compulsion to settle down. Even as a tenured professor who could afford something better, I lived in a

$450-a-month attic apartment with a fire-escape walkup. It was a place my grad students wouldn't live in because it was beneath them. But it was perfect for me.

A friend once asked me: "What kind of woman do you think would be impressed if you brought her back to this place?"

I replied: "The right kind."

But who was I kidding? I was a fun-loving, workaholic Peter Pan with metal folding chairs in my dining room. No woman, even the right kind, would expect to settle down blissfully into that. (And when Jai finally arrived in my life, neither did she.) Granted, I had a good job and other things going for me. But I wasn't any woman's idea of perfect marriage material.

I met Jai in the fall of 1998, when I was invited to give a lecture on virtual reality technology at the University of North Carolina at Chapel Hill. Jai, then a thirty-one-year-old grad student in comparative literature, was working part-time in the UNC computer science department. Her job was to host visitors who came to the labs, whether Nobel laureates or Girl Scout troops. On that particular day, her job was to host me.

Jai had seen me speak the previous summer at a computer graphics conference in Orlando. She later told me she had considered coming up to me afterward to introduce herself, but she never did. When she learned she'd be my host when I came to UNC, she visited my Web site to learn more about me. She clicked through all my academic stuff, and then found

the links to my funkier personal information—that my hob-
bies were making gingerbread houses and sewing. She saw my
age, and no mention of a wife or girlfriend, but lots of photos
of my niece and nephew.

She figured I'm obviously a pretty offbeat and interesting
guy, and she was intrigued enough to make a few phone calls
to friends of hers in the computer science community.

"What do you know about Randy Pausch?" she asked. "Is
he gay?"

She was told I was not. In fact, she was told I had a reputation as a player who'd never settle down (well, to the extent
that a computer scientist can be considered a "player").

As for Jai, she had been married briefly to her college
sweetheart, and after that ended in divorce, with no children,
she was gun-shy about getting serious again.

From the moment I met her the day of my visit, I just
found myself staring at her. She's a beauty, of course, and she
had this gorgeous long hair then, and this smile that said a lot
about both her warmth and her impishness. I was brought
into a lab to watch students demonstrate their virtual reality
projects, and I had trouble concentrating on any of them because Jai was standing there.

Soon enough, I was flirting pretty aggressively. Because
this was a professional setting, that meant I was making far
more eye contact than was appropriate. Jai later told me: "I
couldn't tell if you did that with everyone, or if you were singling me out." Believe me, I was singling.

At one point during the day, Jai sat down with me to ask

questions about bringing software projects to UNC. By then I was completely taken with her. I had to go to a formal faculty dinner that night, but I asked if she'd meet me for a drink afterward. She agreed.

I couldn't concentrate during dinner. I wished all of those tenured professors would just chew faster. I convinced everyone not to order dessert. And I got out of there at 8:30 and called Jai.

We went to a wine bar, even though I don't really drink, and I quickly felt a magnetic sense that I really wanted to be with this woman. I was scheduled to take a flight home the next morning, but I told her I'd change it if she'd go on a date with me the following day. She said yes, and we ended up having a terrific time.

After I returned to Pittsburgh, I offered her my frequent flyer miles and asked her to visit me. She had obvious feelings for me, but she was scared—of both my reputation and of the possibility that she was falling in love.

"I'm not coming," she wrote in an email. "I've thought it through, and I'm not looking for a long-distance relationship. I'm sorry."

I was hooked, of course, and this was a brick wall I thought I could manage. I sent her a dozen roses and a card that read: "Although it saddens me greatly, I respect your decision and wish you nothing but the best. Randy."

Well, that worked. She got on the plane.

I admit: I'm either an incurable romantic or a bit

Machiavellian. But I just wanted her in my life. I *had* fallen in love, even if she was still finding her way.

We saw each other most every weekend through the winter. Though Jai wasn't thrilled with my bluntness and my know-it-all attitude, she said I was the most positive, upbeat person she'd ever met. And she was bringing out good things in me. I found myself caring about her welfare and happiness more than anything else.

Eventually, I asked her to move to Pittsburgh. I offered to get her an engagement ring, but I knew she was still scared and that would freak her out. So I didn't pressure her, and she did agree to a first step: moving up and getting her own apartment.

In April, I made arrangements to teach a weeklong seminar at UNC. That would allow me to help her pack up so we could drive her belongings up to Pittsburgh.

After I arrived in Chapel Hill, Jai told me we needed to talk. She was more serious than I had ever seen her.

"I can't come to Pittsburgh. I'm sorry," she said.

I wondered what was in her head. I asked for an explanation.

Her answer: "This is never going to work." I had to know why.

"I just . . ." she said. "I just don't love you the way you want me to love you." And then again, for emphasis: "I don't love you."

I was horrified and heartbroken. It was like a punch in the gut. Could she really mean that?

It was an awkward scene. She didn't know how to feel. I didn't know how to feel. I needed a ride over to my hotel. "Would you be kind enough to drive me or should I call a cab?"

She drove me, and when we got there, I pulled my bag out of her trunk, fighting back tears. If it's possible to be arrogant, optimistic and totally miserable all at the same time, I think I might have pulled it off: "Look, I'm going to find a way to be happy, and I'd really love to be happy with you, but if I can't be happy with you, then I'll find a way to be happy without you."

In the hotel, I spent much of the day on the phone with my parents, telling them about the brick wall I'd just smashed into. Their advice was incredible.

"Look," my dad said. "I don't think she means it. It's not consistent with her behavior thus far. You've asked her to pull up roots and run away with you. She's probably confused and scared to death. If she doesn't really love you, then it's over. And if she does love you, then love will win out."

I asked my parents what I should do.

"Be supportive," my mom said. "If you love her, support her."

And so I did that. I spent that week teaching, hanging out in an office up the hall from Jai. I stopped by a couple of times, however, just to see if she was all right. "I just wanted to see how you are," I'd say. "If there's anything I can do, let me know."

A few days later, Jai called. "Well, Randy, I'm sitting here missing you, just wishing you were here. That means something, doesn't it?"

She had come to a realization: She was in love, after all. Once again, my parents had come through. Love *had* won out. At week's end, Jai moved to Pittsburgh.

Brick walls are there for a reason. They give us a chance to show how badly we want something.

17

Not All Fairy Tales End Smoothly

J AI AND I were married under a 100-year-old oak tree on the lawn of a famous Victorian mansion in Pittsburgh. It was a small wedding, but I like big romantic statements, and so Jai and I agreed to start our marriage in a special way.

We did not leave the reception in a car with cans rattling from the rear bumper. We did not get into a horse-drawn carriage. Instead, we got into a huge, multicolored hot-air balloon that whisked us off into the clouds, as our friends and loved ones waved up to us, wishing us bon voyage. What a Kodak moment!

When we had stepped into the balloon, Jai was just beaming. "It's like a fairy tale ending to a Disney movie," she said.

Then the balloon smashed through tree branches on the way up. It didn't sound like the destruction of the Hindenburg, but it was a little disconcerting. "No problem," said the man flying the balloon. (He's called a "ballooner.") "Usually we're OK going through branches."

Usually?

We had also taken off a little later than scheduled, and the ballooner said that could make things harder, because it was getting dark. And the winds had shifted. "I can't really control where we go. We're at the mercy of the winds," he said. "But we should be OK."

The balloon traveled over urban Pittsburgh, back and forth above the city's famous three rivers. This was not where the ballooner wanted to be, and I could see he was worried. "There's no place to put this bird down," he said, almost to himself. Then to us: "We've got to keep looking."

The newlyweds were no longer enjoying the view. We were all looking for a large open space hidden in an urban landscape. Finally, we floated into the suburbs, and the ballooner spotted a big field off in the distance. He committed to putting the balloon down in it. "This should work," he said as he started descending fast.

I looked down at the field. It appeared to be fairly large, but I noticed there was a train track at the edge of it. My eyes followed the track. A train was coming. At that moment, I was no longer a groom. I was an engineer. I said to the ballooner: "Sir, I think I see a variable here."

"A variable? Is that what you computer guys call a problem?" he asked.

"Well, yes. What if we hit the train?"

He answered honestly. We were in the basket of the balloon, and the odds of the basket hitting the train were small.

However, there was certainly a risk that the giant balloon itself (called "the envelope") would fall onto the tracks when we hit the ground. If the speeding train got tangled in the falling envelope, we'd be at the wrong end of a rope, inside a basket getting dragged. In that case, great bodily harm was not just possible, but probable.

"When this thing hits the ground, run as fast as you can," the ballooner said. These are not the words most brides dream about hearing on their wedding day. In short, Jai was no longer feeling like a Disney princess. And I was already seeing myself as a character in a disaster movie, thinking of how I'd save my new bride during the calamity apparently to come.

I looked into the eyes of the ballooner. I often rely on people with expertise I don't have, and I wanted to get a clear sense of where he was on this. In his face, I saw more than concern. I saw mild panic. I also saw fear. I looked at Jai. I'd enjoyed our marriage so far.

As the balloon kept descending, I tried to calculate how fast we'd need to jump out of the basket and run for our lives. I figured the ballooner could handle himself, and if not, well, I was still grabbing Jai first. I loved her. Him, I'd just met.

The ballooner kept letting air out of the balloon. He pulled every lever he had. He just wanted to get down somewhere, quickly. At that point, he'd be better off hitting a nearby house than that speeding train.

The basket took a hard hit as we crash-landed in the field,

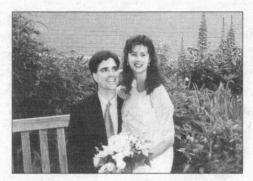

This was taken *before* we got into the balloon.

hopped a few times, bouncing all around, and then tilted almost horizontally. Within seconds, the deflating envelope draped onto the ground. But luckily, it missed the moving train. Meanwhile, people on the nearby highway saw our landing, stopped their cars, and ran to help us. It was quite a scene: Jai in her wedding dress, me in my suit, the collapsed balloon, the relieved ballooner.

We were pretty rattled. My friend Jack had been in the chase car, tracking the balloon from the ground. When he got to us, he was happy to find us safe following our near-death experience.

We spent some time decompressing from our reminder that even fairy-tale moments have risks, while the collapsed balloon was loaded onto the ballooner's truck. Then, just as

Jack was about to take us home, the ballooner came trotting over to us. "Wait, wait!" he said. "You ordered the wedding package! It comes with a bottle of champagne!" He handed us a cheap bottle from his truck. "Congratulations!" he said.

We smiled weakly and thanked him. It was only dusk on our first day of marriage, but we'd made it so far.

18

Lucy, I'm Home

ONE WARM day, early in our marriage, I walked to Carnegie Mellon and Jai was at home. I remember this because that particular day became famous in our household as "The Day Jai Managed to Achieve the One-Driver, Two-Car Collision."

Our minivan was in the garage and my Volkswagen convertible was in the driveway. Jai pulled out the minivan without realizing the other car was in the way. The result: an instantaneous crunch, boom, bam!

What followed just proves that at times we're all living in an *I Love Lucy* episode. Jai spent the entire day obsessing over how to explain everything to Ricky when he got home from Club Babalu.

She thought it best to create the perfect circumstances to break the news. She made sure both cars were in the garage with the garage door closed. She was more sweet than usual when I arrived home, asking me all about my day. She put on soft music. She made me my favorite meal. She wasn't wearing a negligee—I wasn't that lucky—but she did her best to be the perfect, loving partner.

Toward the end of our terrific dinner she said, "Randy, I have something to tell you. I hit one car with the other car."

I asked her how it happened. I had her describe the damage. She said the convertible got the worst of it, but both cars were running fine. "Want to go in the garage and look at them?" she asked.

"No," I said. "Let's just finish dinner."

She was surprised. I wasn't angry. I hardly seemed concerned. As she'd soon learn, my measured response was rooted in my upbringing.

After dinner, we looked at the cars. I just shrugged, and I could see that for Jai, an entire day's worth of anxiety was just melting away. "Tomorrow morning," she promised, "I'll get estimates on the repairs."

I told her that wasn't necessary. The dents would be OK. My parents had raised me to recognize that automobiles are there to get you from point A to point B. They are utilitarian devices, not expressions of social status. And so I told Jai we didn't need to do cosmetic repairs. We'd just live with the dents and gashes.

Jai was a bit shocked. "We're really going to drive around in dented cars?" she asked.

"Well, you can't have just some of me, Jai," I told her. "You appreciate the part of me that didn't get angry because two 'things' we own got hurt. But the flip side of that is my belief that you don't repair things if they still do what they're supposed to do. The cars still work. Let's just drive 'em."

OK, maybe this makes me quirky. But if your trashcan or wheelbarrow has a dent in it, you don't buy a new one. Maybe that's because we don't use trashcans and wheelbarrows to communicate our social status or identity to others. For Jai and me, our dented cars became a statement in our marriage. Not everything needs to be fixed.

19

A New Year's Story

No matter how bad things are, you can always make things worse. At the same time, it is often within your power to make them better. I learned this lesson well on New Year's Eve 2001.

Jai was seven months pregnant with Dylan, and we were about to welcome in 2002 having a quiet night at home, watching a DVD.

The movie was just starting when Jai said, "I think my water just broke." But it wasn't water. It was blood. Within an instant, she was bleeding so profusely that I realized there was no time to even call an ambulance. Pittsburgh's Magee-Womens Hospital was four minutes away if I ignored red lights, which is what I did.

When we got to the emergency room, doctors, nurses and other hospital personnel descended with IVs, stethoscopes and insurance forms. It was quickly determined that her placenta had torn away from the uterine wall; it's called "placenta abrupta." With the placenta in such distress, the life support for the fetus was giving out. They don't need to tell you how serious this is. Jai's health and the viability of our baby were at great risk.

For weeks, the pregnancy hadn't been going smoothly. Jai could hardly feel the baby kicking. She wasn't gaining enough weight. Knowing how crucial it is for people to be aggressive about their medical care, I had insisted that she be given another ultrasound. That's when doctors realized Jai's placenta wasn't operating efficiently. The baby wasn't thriving. And so doctors gave Jai a steroid shot to stimulate the development of the baby's lungs.

It was all worrisome. But now, here in the emergency room, things had gotten far more serious.

"Your wife is approaching clinical shock," a nurse said. Jai was so scared. I saw that on her face. How was I? Also scared, but I was trying to remain calm so I could assess the situation.

I looked around me. It was 9 p.m. on New Year's Eve. Surely, any doctor or nurse on the hospital's seniority list had gotten off for the night. I had to assume this was the B team. Would they be up to the job of saving my child and my wife?

It did not take long, however, for these doctors and nurses to impress me. If they were the B team, they were awfully good. They took over with a wonderful mix of hurry and calm. They didn't seem panicked. They carried themselves like they knew how to efficiently do what had to be done, moment by moment. And they *said* all the right things.

As Jai was being rushed into surgery for an emergency C-section, she said to the doctor, "This is bad, isn't it?"

I admired the doctor's response. It was the perfect answer for our times: "If we were really in a panic, we wouldn't have had you sign all the insurance forms, would we?" she said to Jai. "We wouldn't have taken the time." The doctor had a point. I wondered how often she used her "hospital paper-work" riff to ease patients' anxieties.

Whatever the case, her words helped. And then the anesthesiologist took me aside.

"Look, you're going to have a job tonight," he said, "and you're the only person who can do it. Your wife is halfway to clinical shock. If she goes into shock, we can treat her. But it won't be easy for us. So you have to help her remain calm. We want you to keep her with us."

So often, everyone pretends that husbands have an actual role when babies are born. "Breathe, honey. Good. Keep breathing. Good." My dad always found that coaching culture amusing, since he was out having cheeseburgers when his first child was born. But now I was being given a real job. The anesthesiologist was straightforward, but I sensed the intensity of his request. "I don't know what you should say to her or how you should say it," he told me. "I'll trust you to figure that out. Just keep her off the ledge when she gets scared."

They began the C-section and I held Jai's hand as tightly as I could. I was able to see what was going on and she couldn't. I decided I would calmly tell her everything that was happening. I'd give her the truth.

Her lips were blue. She was shaking. I was rubbing her head, then holding her hand with both of mine, trying to describe the surgery in a way that was direct yet reassuring. For her part, Jai tried desperately to remain with us, to stay calm and conscious.

"I see a baby," I said. "There's a baby coming."

Through tears, she couldn't ask the hardest question. But I had the answer. "He's moving."

And then the baby, our first child, Dylan, let out a wail like you've never heard before. Just bloody murder. The nurses smiled. "That's great," someone said. The preemies who come out limp often have the most trouble. But the ones who come out all pissed off and full of noise, they're the fighters. They're the ones who thrive.

Dylan weighed two pounds, fifteen ounces. His head was about the size of a baseball. But the good news was that he was breathing well on his own.

Jai was overcome with emotion and relief. In her smile, I saw her blue lips fading back toward normal. I was so proud of her. Her courage amazed me. Had I kept her from going into shock? I don't know. But I had tried to say and do and feel everything possible to keep her with us. I had tried not to panic. Maybe it had helped.

Dylan was sent to the neonatal intensive care unit. I came to recognize that parents with babies there needed very specific reassurances from doctors and nurses. At Magee, they did a wonderful job of simultaneously communicating two dissonant things. In so many words, they told parents that

1) Your child is special and we understand that his medical needs are unique, and 2) Don't worry, we've had a million babies like yours come through here.

Dylan never needed a respirator, but day after day, we still felt this intense fear that he could take a downward turn. It just felt too early to fully celebrate our new three-person family. When Jai and I drove to the hospital each day, there was an unspoken thought in both our heads: "Will our baby be alive when we get there?"

One day, we arrived at the hospital and Dylan's bassinette was gone. Jai almost collapsed from emotion. My heart was pounding. I grabbed the nearest nurse, literally by the lapels, and I couldn't even pull together complete sentences. I was gasping out fear in staccato.

"Baby. Last name Pausch. Where?"

In that moment, I felt drained in a way I can't quite explain. I feared I was about to enter a dark place I'd never been invited to before.

But the nurse just smiled. "Oh, your baby is doing so well that we moved him upstairs to an open-air bassinette," she said. He'd been in a so-called "closed-air bassinette," which is a more benign description of an incubator.

In relief, we raced up the stairs to the other ward, and there was Dylan, screaming his way into his childhood.

Dylan's birth was a reminder to me of the roles we get to play in our destinies. Jai and I could have made things worse by falling into pieces. She could have gotten so hysterical that she'd thrown herself into shock. I could have been so stricken that I'd have been no help in the operating room.

Through the whole ordeal, I don't think we ever said to each other: "This isn't fair." We just kept going. We recognized that there *were* things we could do that might help the outcome in positive ways . . . and we did them. Without saying it in words, our attitude was, "Let's saddle up and ride."

20

"In Fifty Years, It Never Came Up"

AFTER MY father passed away in 2006, we went through his things. He was always so full of life and his belongings spoke of his adventures. I found photos of him as a young man playing an accordion, as a middle-aged man dressed in a Santa suit (he loved playing Santa), and as an older man, clutching a stuffed bear bigger than he was. In another photo, taken on his eightieth birthday, he was riding a roller coaster with a bunch of twentysomethings, and he had this great grin on his face.

In my dad's things, I came upon mysteries that made me smile. My dad had a photo of himself—it looks like it was taken in the early 1960s—and he was in a jacket and tie, in a grocery store. In one hand, he held up a small brown paper bag. I'll never know what was in that bag, but knowing my father, it had to be something cool.

After work, he'd sometimes bring home a small toy or a piece of candy, and he'd present them with a flourish, building a bit of drama. His delivery was more fun than whatever he had for us. That's what that bag photo brought to my mind.

My dad had also saved a stack of papers. There were letters regarding his insurance business and documents about his charitable projects. Then, buried in the stack, we found a

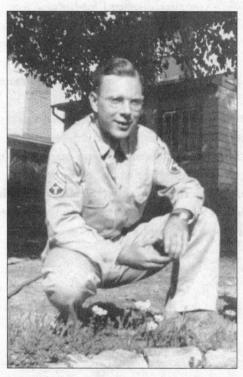

My father, in uniform.

citation issued in 1945, when my father was in the army. The citation for "heroic achievement" came from the commanding general of the 75th Infantry Division.

On April 11, 1945, my father's infantry company was attacked by German forces, and in the early stages of battle, heavy artillery fire led to eight casualties. According to the citation: "With complete disregard for his own safety, Private Pausch leaped from a covered position and commenced treating the wounded men while shells continued to fall in the immediate vicinity. So successfully did this soldier administer medical attention that all the wounded were evacuated successfully."

In recognition of this, my dad, then twenty-two years old, was issued the Bronze Star for valor.

In the fifty years my parents were married, in the thousands of conversations my dad had with me, it had just never come up. And so there I was, weeks after his death, getting another lesson from him about the meaning of sacrifice—and about the power of humility.

21

Jai

I'VE ASKED Jai what she has learned since my diagnosis. Turns out, she could write a book titled *Forget the Last Lecture; Here's the Real Story.*

She's a strong woman, my wife. I admire her directness, her honesty, her willingness to tell it to me straight. Even now, with just months to go, we try to interact with each other as if everything is normal and our marriage has decades to go. We discuss, we get frustrated, we get mad, we make up.

Jai says she's still figuring out how to deal with me, but she's making headway.

"You're always the scientist, Randy," she says. "You want science? I'll give you science." She used to tell me she had "a gut feeling" about something. Now, instead, she brings me data.

For instance, we were going to visit my side of the family over this past Christmas, but they all had the flu. Jai didn't want to expose me or our kids to the chance of infection. I thought we should take the trip. After all, I won't have many more opportunities to see my family.

"We'll all keep our distance," I said. "We'll be fine."

Jai knew she'd need data. She called a friend who is a nurse. She called two doctors who lived up the street. She got their medical opinions. They said it wouldn't be smart to take the kids. "I've got unbiased third-party medical authorities, Randy," she said. "Here's their input." Presented with the data, I relented. I went for a quick trip to see my family and Jai stayed home with the kids. (I didn't get the flu.)

I know what you're thinking. Scientists like me probably aren't always easy to live with.

Jai handles me by being frank. When I've gone off course, she lets me know. Or she gives me a warning: "Something is bugging me. I don't know what it is. When I figure it out, I'll tell you."

At the same time, given my prognosis, Jai says she's learning to let some of the little stuff slide. That's a suggestion from our counselor. Dr. Reiss has a gift for helping people recalibrate their home lives when one spouse has a terminal illness. Marriages like ours have to find their way to "a new normal."

I'm a spreader. My clothes, clean and dirty, are spread around the bedroom, and my bathroom sink is cluttered. It drives Jai crazy. Before I got sick, she'd say something. But Dr. Reiss has advised her not to let small things trip us up.

Obviously, I ought to be neater. I owe Jai many apologies. But she has stopped telling me about the minor stuff that bugs her. Do we really want to spend our last months together arguing that I haven't hung up my khakis? We do not. So now Jai kicks my clothes into a corner and moves on.

A friend of ours suggested that Jai keep a daily journal, and Jai says it helps. She writes in there the things that get on her nerves about me. "Randy didn't put his plate in the dishwasher tonight," she wrote one night. "He just left it there on the table, and went to his computer." She knew I was preoccupied, heading to the Internet to research possible medical treatments. Still, the dish on the table bothered her. I can't blame her. So she wrote about it, felt better, and again we didn't have to get into an argument.

Jai tries to focus on each day, rather than the negative things down the road. "It's not helpful if we spend every day dreading tomorrow," she says.

This last New Year's Eve, though, was very emotional and bittersweet in our house. It was Dylan's sixth birthday, so there was a celebration. We also were grateful that I had made it to the new year. But we couldn't bring ourselves to discuss the elephant in the room: the future New Year's Eves without me.

I took Dylan to see a movie that day, *Mr. Magorium's Wonder Emporium,* about a toymaker. I had read an online description of the film, but it didn't mention that Mr. Magorium had decided it was time to die and hand over the shop to an apprentice. So there I was in the theater, with Dylan on my lap, and he was crying about how Mr. Magorium was dying. (Dylan doesn't yet know my prognosis.) If my life were a movie, this scene of me and Dylan would get slammed by critics for over-the-top foreshadowing. There was one line in the film, however, that remains with me. The apprentice

(Natalie Portman) tells the toymaker (Dustin Hoffman) that he can't die; he has to live. And he responds: "I already did that."

Later that night, as the new year approached, Jai could tell I was depressed. To cheer me up, she reviewed the past year and pointed out some of the wonderful things that had happened. We had gone on romantic vacations, just the two of us, that we wouldn't have taken if cancer hadn't offered a reminder about the preciousness of time. We had watched the kids grow into their own; our house was really filled with a beautiful energy and a great deal of love.

Jai vowed she'd continue to be there for me and the kids. "I have four very good reasons to suck it up and keep going. And I will," she promised.

Jai also told me that one of the best parts of her day is watching me interact with the kids. She says my face lights up when Chloe talks to me. (Chloe is eighteen months old and is already talking in four-word sentences.)

At Christmas, I had made an adventure out of putting the lights on the tree. Rather than showing Dylan and Logan the proper way to do it—carefully and meticulously—I just let them have at it haphazardly. However they wanted to throw those lights on the tree was fine by me. We got video of the whole chaotic scene, and Jai says it was a "magical moment" that will be one of her favorite memories of our family together.

* * *

Jai has gone on Web sites for cancer patients and their families. She finds useful information there, but she can't stay on too long. "So many of the entries begin: 'Bob's fight is over.' 'Jim's fight is over.' I don't think it's helpful to keep reading all of that," she says.

However, one entry she came upon moved her into action. It was written by a woman whose husband had pancreatic cancer. They planned to take a family vacation but postponed it. He died before they could reschedule. "Go on those trips you've always wanted to take," the woman advised other caregivers. "Live in the moment." Jai vows to keep doing just that.

Jai has gotten to know people locally who are also caregivers of spouses with terminal illnesses, and she finds it helpful to talk to them. If she needs to complain about me, or to vent about the pressure she's under, these conversations have been a good outlet for her.

At the same time, she tries to focus on our happiest times. When I was courting her, I sent her flowers once a week. I hung stuffed animals in her office. I went overboard, and—when I wasn't scaring her off—she enjoyed it! Lately, she says, she'd been pulling up her memories of Randy the Romantic, and that makes her smile and helps her get through her down moments.

Jai, by the way, has lived out a good number of her childhood dreams. She wanted to own a horse. (That never happened, but she has done a lot of riding.) She wanted to go to France. (That happened; she lived in France one summer in college.) And most of all, she dreamed as a girl of having children of her own someday.

I wish I had more time to help her realize other dreams.

But the kids are a spectacular dream fulfilled, and there's great solace in that for both of us.

When Jai and I talk about the lessons she has learned from our journey, she talks about how we've found strength in standing together, shoulder to shoulder. She says she's grateful that we can talk, heart to heart. And then she tells me about how my clothes are all over the room and it's very annoying, but she's giving me a pass, all things considered. I know: Before she starts scribbling in her journal, I owe it to her to straighten up my mess. I'll try harder. It's one of my New Year's resolutions.

22

The Truth Can Set You Free

—————

I RECENTLY GOT pulled over for speeding not far from my new home in Virginia. I hadn't been paying attention, and I had drifted a few miles an hour over the speed limit.

"Can I see your license and registration?" the police officer asked me. I pulled both out for him, and he saw my Pittsburgh address on my Pennsylvania driver's license.

"What are you doing here?" he asked. "You with the military?"

"No, I'm not," I said. I explained that I had just moved to Virginia, and I hadn't had time to re-register yet.

"So what brings you here?"

He had asked a direct question. Without thinking very hard, I gave him a direct answer. "Well, officer," I said, "since you've asked, I have terminal cancer. I have just months to live. We've moved down here to be close to my wife's family."

The officer cocked his head and squinted at me. "So you've got cancer," he said flatly. He was trying to figure me out. Was I really dying? Was I lying? He took a long look at me. "You know, for a guy who has only a few months to live, you sure look good."

He was obviously thinking: "Either this guy is pulling one big fat line on me, or he's telling the truth. And I have no way of knowing." This wasn't an easy encounter for him because he was trying to do the near-impossible. He was trying to question my integrity without directly calling me a liar. And so he had forced me to prove that I was being honest. How would I do that?

"Well, officer, I know that I look pretty healthy. It's really ironic. I look great on the outside, but the tumors are on the inside." And then, I don't know what possessed me, but I just did it. I pulled up my shirt, revealing the surgical scars.

The cop looked at my scars. He looked in my eyes. I could see on his face: He now knew he was talking to a dying man. And if by some chance I was the most brazen con man he'd ever stopped, well, he wasn't taking this any further. He handed me back my license. "Do me a favor," he said. "Slow down from now on."

The awful truth had set me free. As he trotted back to his police car, I had a realization. I have never been one of those gorgeous blondes who could bat her eyelashes and get out of tickets. I drove home under the speed limit, and I was smiling like a beauty queen.

IV

ENABLING THE DREAMS OF OTHERS

23

I'm on My Honeymoon,
But If You Need Me . . .

———————

JAI SENT me out to buy a few groceries the other day. After I found everything on the list, I figured I'd get out of the store faster if I used the self-scan aisle. I slid my credit card into the machine, followed the directions, and scanned my groceries myself. The machine chirped, beeped and said I owed $16.55, but issued no receipt. So I swiped my credit card again and started over.

Soon, two receipts popped out. The machine had charged me twice.

At that point, I had a decision to make. I could have tracked down the manager, who would have listened to my story, filled out some form, and taken my credit card to his register to remove one of the $16.55 charges. The whole tedious ordeal could have stretched to ten or even fifteen minutes. It would have been zero fun for me.

Given my short road ahead, did I want to spend those precious minutes getting that refund? I did not. Could I afford to pay the extra $16.55? I could. So I left the store, happier to have fifteen minutes than sixteen dollars.

All my life, I've been very aware that time is finite. I admit I'm overly logical about a lot of things, but I firmly believe that one of my most appropriate fixations has been to manage time well. I've railed about time management to my students. I've given lectures on it. And because I've gotten so good at it, I really do feel I was able to pack a whole lot of life into the shortened lifespan I've been handed.

Here's what I know:

Time must be explicitly managed, like money. My students would sometimes roll their eyes at what they called "Pauschisms," but I stand by them. Urging students not to invest time on irrelevant details, I'd tell them: "It doesn't matter how well you polish the underside of the banister."

You can always change your plan, but only if you have one. I'm a big believer in to-do lists. It helps us break life into small steps. I once put "get tenure" on my to-do list. That was naïve. The most useful to-do list breaks tasks into small steps. It's like when I encourage Logan to clean his room by picking up one thing at a time.

Ask yourself: Are you spending your time on the right things? You may have causes, goals, interests. Are they even worth pursuing? I've long held on to a clipping from a newspaper in Roanoke, Virginia. It featured a photo of a pregnant woman who had lodged a protest against a local construction site. She worried that the sound of jackhammers was injuring her unborn child. But get this: In the photo, the woman is holding a cigarette. If she cared about her unborn child, the time she spent railing against jackhammers would have been better spent putting out that cigarette.

Develop a good filing system. When I told Jai I wanted to have a place in the house where we could file everything in alphabetical order, she said I sounded way too compulsive for her tastes. I told her: "Filing in alphabetical order is better than running around and saying, 'I know it was blue and I know I was eating something when I had it.'"

Rethink the telephone. I live in a culture where I spend a lot of time on hold, listening to "Your call is very important to us." Yeah, right. That's like a guy slapping a girl in the face on a first date and saying, "I actually do love you." Yet that's how modern customer service works. And I reject that. I make sure I am never on hold with a phone against my ear. I always use a speaker phone, so my hands are free to do something else.

I've also collected techniques for keeping unnecessary calls shorter. If I'm sitting while on the phone, I never put my feet up. In fact, it's better to stand when you're on the phone. You're more apt to speed things along. I also like to have something in view on my desk that I want to do, so I have the urge to wrap things up with the caller.

Over the years, I've picked up other phone tips. Want to quickly dispatch telemarketers? Hang up while you're doing the talking and they're listening. They'll assume your connection went bad and they'll move on to their next call. Want to have a short phone call with someone? Call them at 11:55 a.m., right before lunch. They'll talk fast. You may think you are interesting, but you are not more interesting than lunch.

Delegate. As a professor, I learned early on that I could trust bright, nineteen-year-old students with the keys to my kingdom, and most of the time, they were responsible and impressive. It's never too early to delegate. My daughter, Chloe, is just eighteen months old, but two of my favorite photos are of her in my arms. In the first, I'm giving her a bottle. In the second, I've delegated the task to her. She looks satisfied. Me, too.

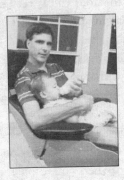 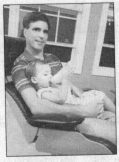

Take a time out. It's not a real vacation if you're reading email or calling in for messages. When Jai and I went on our honeymoon, we wanted to be left alone. My boss, however, felt I needed to provide a way for people to contact me. So I came up with the perfect phone message:

"Hi, this is Randy. I waited until I was thirty-nine to get married, so my wife and I are going away for a month. I hope you don't have a problem with that, but my boss does. Apparently, I have to be reachable." I then gave the names of Jai's parents and the city where they live. "If you call directory assistance, you can get their number. And then, if you can convince my new in-laws that your emergency merits interrupting their only daughter's honeymoon, they have our number."

We didn't get any calls.

Some of my time management tips are dead-on serious and some are a bit tongue-in-cheek. But I believe all of them are worth considering.

Time is all you have. And you may find one day that you have less than you think.

24

A Recovering Jerk

I T IS an accepted cliché in education that the number one
goal of teachers should be to help students learn how to
learn.

I always saw the value in that, sure. But in my mind, a better number one goal was this: I wanted to help students learn
how to judge themselves.

Did they recognize their true abilities? Did they have a
sense of their own flaws? Were they realistic about how others
viewed them?

In the end, educators best serve students by helping them
be more self-reflective. The only way any of us can
improve—as Coach Graham taught me—is if we develop a
real ability to assess ourselves. If we can't accurately do that,
how can we tell if we're getting better or worse?

Some old-school types complain these days that higher education too often feels like it is all about customer service.
Students and their parents believe they are paying top dollar
for a product, and so they want it to be valuable in a measur-

able way. It's as if they've walked into a department store, and instead of buying five pairs of designer jeans, they've purchased a five-subject course-load.

I don't fully reject the customer-service model, but I think it's important to use the right industry metaphor. It's not retail. Instead, I'd compare college tuition to paying for a personal trainer at an athletic club. We professors play the roles of trainers, giving people access to the equipment (books, labs, our expertise) and after that, it is our job to be demanding. We need to make sure that our students are exerting themselves. We need to praise them when they deserve it and to tell them honestly when they have it in them to work harder.

Most importantly, we need to let them know how to judge for themselves how they're coming along. The great thing about working out at a gym is that if you put in effort, you get very obvious results. The same should be true of college. A professor's job is to teach students how to see their minds growing in the same way they can see their muscles grow when they look in a mirror.

To that end, I've tried hard to come up with mechanical ways to get people to listen to feedback. I was constantly helping my students develop their own feedback loops. It was not easy. Getting people to welcome feedback was the hardest thing I ever had to do as an educator. (It hasn't been easy in my personal life, either.) It saddens me that so many parents and educators have given up on this. When they talk of building self-esteem, they often resort to empty flattery rather than character-building honesty. I've heard so many people talk of a downward spiral in our educational system, and I think one key factor is that there is too much stroking and too little real feedback.

When I taught the "Building Virtual Worlds" class at Carnegie Mellon, we'd do peer feedback every two weeks. This was a completely collaborative class, with the students working in four-person teams on virtual-reality computer projects. They were dependent on each other, and their grades reflected it.

We would take all of the peer feedback and put together a spreadsheet. At the end of the semester, after each student had worked on five projects, with three different teammates on each, everyone would have fifteen data points. That was a pragmatic, statistically valid way to look at themselves.

I would create multicolored bar charts in which a student could see a ranking on simple measures such as:

1) Did his peers think he was working hard? Exactly how many hours did his peers think he had devoted to a project?
2) How creative was his contribution?
3) Did his peers find it easy or hard to work with him? Was he a team player?

As I always pointed out, especially for No. 3, what your peers think is, by definition, an accurate assessment of how easy you are to work with.

The multicolored bar charts were very specific. All the students knew where they stood relative to their forty-nine peers.

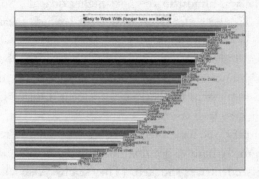

The bar charts were coupled with more free-form peer feedback, which was essentially specific suggestions for improvement, such as "Let other people finish their sentences when they're talking."

My hope was that more than a few students would see this information and say, "Wow, I've got to take it up a notch." It was hard feedback to ignore, but some still managed.

For one course I taught, I'd had students assess each other in the same way, but only let them know the quartile in which they ranked. I remember a conversation I had with one student whom others found particularly obnoxious. He was smart, but his healthy sense of himself left him clueless about how he was coming off. He saw the data ranking him in the bottom quartile and remained unfazed.

He figured that if he was ranked in the bottom 25 percent, he must have been at the 24 percent or 25 percent level (rather than, say, in the bottom 5 percent). So in his mind, that meant he was almost in the next higher quartile. So he saw himself as "not so far from 50 percent," which meant peers thought he was just fine.

"I'm so glad we had this chat," I told him, "because I think it's important that I give you some specific information. You are not just in the bottom 25 percent. Out of fifty students in the class, your peers ranked you dead last. You are number fifty. You have a serious issue. They say you're not listening. You're hard to get along with. It's not going well."

The student was shocked. (They're always shocked.) He had had all of these rationalizations, and now here I was, giving him hard data.

And then I told him the truth about myself.

"I used to be just like you," I said. "I was in denial. But I had a professor who showed he cared about me by smacking the truth into my head. And here's what makes me special: I listened."

This student's eyes widened. "I admit it," I told him. "I'm a recovering jerk. And that gives me the moral authority to tell you that you can be a recovering jerk, too."

For the rest of the semester, this student kept himself in check. He improved. I'd done him a favor, just as Andy van Dam had done for me years before.

25
Training a Jedi

I T'S A thrill to fulfill your own childhood dreams, but as you get older, you may find that enabling the dreams of others is even more fun.

When I was teaching at the University of Virginia in 1993, a twenty-two-year-old artist-turned-computer-graphics-wiz named Tommy Burnett wanted a job on my research team. After we talked about his life and goals, he suddenly said, "Oh, and I have always had this childhood dream."

Anyone who uses "childhood" and "dream" in the same sentence usually gets my attention.

"And what is your dream, Tommy?" I asked.

"I want to work on the next *Star Wars* film," he said.

Remember, this was in 1993. The last *Star Wars* movie had been made in 1983, and there were no concrete plans to make any more. I explained this. "That's a tough dream to have because it'll be hard to see it through," I told him. "Word is that they're finished making *Star Wars* films."

"No," he said, "they're going to make more, and when they do, I'm going to work on them. That's my plan."

Tommy was six years old when the first *Star Wars* came out in 1977. "Other kids wanted to be Han Solo," he told me. "Not me. I wanted to be the guy who made the special effects—the space ships, the planets, the robots."

He told me that as a boy, he read the most technical *Star Wars* articles he could find. He had all the books that explained how the models were built, and how the special effects were achieved.

As Tommy spoke, I had a flashback to my childhood visit to Disneyland, and how I had this visceral urge to grow up and create those kinds of rides. I figured Tommy's big dream would never happen, but it might serve him well somehow. I could use a dreamer like that. I knew from my NFL desires that even if he didn't achieve his, they could serve him well, so I asked him to join our research team.

Tommy will tell you I was a pretty tough boss. As he now recalls it, I rode him hard and had very high expectations, but he also knew I had his best interests at heart. He compares me to a demanding football coach. (I guess I was channeling Coach Graham.) Tommy also says that he learned not just about virtual reality programming from me, but also about how work colleagues need to be like a family of sorts. He remembers me telling him: "I know you're smart. But everyone here is smart. Smart isn't enough. The kind of people I want on my research team are those who will help everyone else feel happy to be here."

Tommy turned out to be just that kind of team player. After I got tenure, I brought Tommy and others on my research team down to Disney World as a way of saying thanks.

When I moved on to Carnegie Mellon, every member of my team from the University of Virginia came with me—everyone except Tommy. He couldn't make the move. Why? Because he had been hired by producer/director George Lucas's company, Industrial Light & Magic. And it's worth noting that they didn't hire him for his dream; they hired him for his skills. In his time with our research group, he had become an outstanding programmer in the Python language, which as luck would have it, was the language of choice in their shop. Luck is indeed where preparation meets opportunity.

It's not hard to guess where this story is going. Three new *Star Wars* films would be made—in 1999, 2002, and 2005—and Tommy would end up working on all of them.

On *Star Wars Episode II: Attack of the Clones,* Tommy was a lead technical director. There was an incredible fifteen-minute battle scene on a rocky red planet, pitting clones against droids, and Tommy was the guy who planned it all out. He and his team used photos of the Utah desert to create a virtual landscape for the battle. Talk about cool jobs. Tommy had one that let him spend each day on another planet.

A few years later, he was gracious enough to welcome me and my students on a visit to Industrial Light & Magic. My colleague Don Marinelli had started an awesome tradition of taking students on a trip out west every year, so they could check out entertainment and high-tech companies that might give them a start in the world of computer graphics. By then, a guy like Tommy was a god to these students. He was living their dreams.

Tommy sat on a panel with three other former students of mine, and my current students asked questions. This particular bunch of current students was still unsure what to make of me. I'd been my usual self—a tough teacher with high expectations and some quirky ways—and they weren't at the point where they appreciated that. I'm a bit of an acquired taste in that sense, and after only one semester, some were still noticeably wary of me.

The discussion turned to how hard it was to get a first break in the movie business, and someone wanted to know about the role of luck. Tommy volunteered to answer that question. "It does take a lot of luck," he said. "But all of you are already lucky. Getting to work with Randy and learn from him, that's some kind of luck right there. I wouldn't be here if not for Randy."

I'm a guy who has floated in zero gravity. But I was floating even higher that day. I was incredibly appreciative that Tommy felt I helped enable his dreams. But what made it really special was that he was returning the favor by enabling the dreams of my current students (and helping me in the process). That moment turned out to be a turning point in my relationship with that class. Because Tommy was passing it on.

26

They Just Blew Me Away

PEOPLE WHO know me say I'm an efficiency freak. Obviously, they have me pegged. I'd always rather be doing two useful things at once, or better yet, three. That's why, as my teaching career progressed, I started to ponder this question:

If I could help individual students, one on one, as they worked toward achieving their childhood dreams, was there was a way to do it on a larger scale?

I found that larger scale after I arrived at Carnegie Mellon in 1997 as an associate professor of computer science. My specialty was "human-computer interaction," and I created a course called "Building Virtual Worlds," or BVW for short.

The premise was not so far removed from the Mickey Rooney/Judy Garland idea of "Let's put on a show," only it was updated for the age of computer graphics, 3-D animation and the construction of what we called "immersive (helmet-based) interactive virtual reality worlds."

I opened the course to fifty undergraduates from all different departments of the university. We had actors, English majors and sculptors mixed with engineers, math majors and computer geeks. These were students whose paths might never have had reason to cross, given how autonomous the various disciplines at Carnegie Mellon could be. But we made these kids unlikely partners with each other, forcing them to do together what they couldn't do alone.

There were four people per team, randomly chosen, and they remained together for projects that lasted two weeks. I'd just tell them: "Build a virtual world." And so they'd program something, dream up something, show everyone else, and then I'd reshuffle the teams, and they'd get three new play-mates and start again.

I had just two rules for their virtual reality worlds: No shooting violence and no pornography. I issued that decree mostly because those things have been done in computer games only about a zillion times, and I was looking for origi-nal thinking.

You'd be amazed at how many nineteen-year-old boys are completely out of ideas when you take sex and violence off the table. And yet, when I asked them to think far beyond the ob-vious, most of them rose to the challenge. In fact, the first year I offered the course, the students presented their initial projects and they just blew me away. Their work was literally beyond my imagination. I was especially impressed because they were programming on weak computers by Hollywood's virtual reality standards, and they turned out these incredible gems.

I had been a professor for a decade at that point, and when I started BVW, I didn't know what to expect. I gave the first two-week assignment, and ended up being overwhelmed by the results. I didn't know what to do next. I was so at sea that I called my mentor, Andy van Dam.

"Andy, I just gave my students a two-week assignment and they came back and did stuff that, had I given them an entire semester to complete it, I would have given them all A's. What do I do?"

Andy thought for a minute and said: "OK. Here's what you do. Go back into class tomorrow, look them in the eyes and say, 'Guys, that was pretty good, but I know you can do better.'"

His answer left me stupefied. But I followed his advice and it turned out to be exactly right. He was telling me I obviously didn't know how high the bar should be, and I'd only do them a disservice by putting it anywhere.

And the students did keep improving, inspiring me with their creations. Many projects were just brilliant, ranging from you-are-there white-water rafting adventures to romantic gondola trips through Venice to rollerskating ninjas. Some of my students created completely unlikely existential worlds populated by lovable 3-D creatures they first dreamed about as kids.

On show-and-tell days, I'd come to class and in the room would be my fifty students and another fifty people I didn't recognize—roommates, friends, parents. I'd never had parents come to class before! And it snowballed from there. We ended up having such large crowds on presentation days that we had to move into a large auditorium. It would be standing room only, with more than four hundred people cheering for their favorite virtual-reality presentations. Carnegie Mellon's president, Jared Cohon, once told me that it felt like an Ohio State pep rally, except it was about academics.

On presentation days, I always knew which projects would be the best. I could tell by the body language. If students in a particular group were standing close together, I knew they had bonded, and that the virtual world they created would be something worth seeing.

What I most loved about all of this was that teamwork was so central to its success. How far could these students go? I had no idea. Could they fulfill their dreams? The only sure answer I had for that one was, "In this course, you can't do it alone."

* * *

Was there a way to take what we were doing up a notch?

Drama professor Don Marinelli and I, with the university's blessing, made this thing out of whole cloth that was absolutely insane. It was, and is still, called "The Entertainment Technology Center" (www.etc.cmu.edu), but we liked to think of it as "the dream-fulfillment factory": a two-year master's degree program in which artists and technologists came together to work on amusement rides, computer games, animatronics, and anything else they could dream up.

The sane universities never went near this stuff, but Carnegie Mellon gave us explicit license to break the mold.

The two of us personified the mix of arts and technology; right brain/left brain, drama guy/computer guy. Given how different Don and I were, at times we became each other's brick walls. But we always managed to find a way to make things work. The result was that students often got the best of our divergent approaches (and they *certainly* got role models on how to work with people different from themselves). The mix of freedom and teamwork made the feeling in the building absolutely electric. Companies rapidly found out about us, and were actually offering written three-year commitments to hire our students, which meant they were promising to hire people we hadn't even admitted yet.

Don did 70 percent of the work on the ETC and deserves more than 70 percent of the credit. He has also created a satellite campus in Australia, with plans for other campuses in Korea and Singapore. Hundreds of students I'll never know, all over the world, will be able to fulfill their craziest childhood dreams. That feels great.

27

The Promised Land

ENABLING THE dreams of others can be done on several different scales. You can do it one on one, the way I worked with Tommy, the *Star Wars* dreamer. You can do it with fifty or a hundred people at a time, the way we did in the Building Virtual Worlds class or at the ETC. And, if you have large ambitions and a measure of chutzpah, you can attempt to do it on a grand scale, trying to enable the dreams of millions of people.

I'd like to think that's the story of Alice, the Carnegie Mellon software teaching tool I was lucky enough to help develop. Alice allows introductory computing students—and anyone else, young or old—to easily create animations for telling a story, playing an interactive game or making a video. It uses 3-D graphics and drag-and-drop techniques to give users a more engaging, less frustrating first programming experience. Alice is offered free as a public service by Carnegie Mellon, and more than a million people have downloaded it. In the years ahead, usage is expected to soar.

To me, Alice is infinitely scalable. It's scalable to the point where I can picture tens of millions of kids using it to chase their dreams.

From the time we started Alice in the early 1990s, I've loved that it teaches computer programming by use of the head fake. Remember the head fake? That's when you teach somebody something by having them think they're learning something else. So students think they're using Alice to make movies or create video games. The head fake is that they're actually learning how to become computer programmers.

Walt Disney's dream for Disney World was that it would never be finished. He wanted it to keep growing and changing forever. In the same way, I am thrilled that future versions of Alice now being developed by my colleagues will be even better than what we've done in the past. In upcoming iterations, people will think they're writing movie scripts, but they'll actually be learning the Java programming language. And, thanks to my pal Steve Seabolt at Electronic Arts, we've gotten the OK to use characters from the bestselling personal computer video game in history, "The Sims." How cool is that?

I know the project is in terrific hands. Alice's lead designer is Dennis Cosgrove, who was a student of mine at the University of Virginia. Another former student who became a colleague is Caitlin Kelleher. She looked at "Alice" in its earliest stages and said to me, "I know this makes programming easier, but why is it fun?" I replied: "Well, I'm a compulsive male and I like to make little toy soldiers move around on my command, and that's fun."

So Caitlin wondered how Alice could be made just as fun for girls, and figured storytelling was the secret to getting them interested. For her PhD dissertation, she built a system called "Storytelling Alice."

Now a computer science professor at Washington University in St. Louis, Caitlin (oops, I mean, Dr. Kelleher) is developing new systems that revolutionize how young girls get their first programming experiences. She demonstrated that if it is presented as a storytelling activity, girls become perfectly willing to learn how to write software. In fact, they love it. It's also worth noting that it in no way turns the boys off. Everybody loves telling stories. It's one of the truly universal things about our species. So in my mind, Caitlin wins the All-Time Best Head-Fake Award.

In my last lecture, I mentioned that I now have a better understanding of the story of Moses, and how he got to see the Promised Land but never got to set foot in it. I feel that way about all the successes ahead for Alice.

I wanted my lecture to be a call to my colleagues and students to go on without me, and to know I have confidence that they will do great things. (You can keep tabs on their progress at www.alice.org.)

Through Alice, millions of kids are going to have incredible fun while learning something hard. They'll develop skills that could help them achieve their dreams. If I have to die, I am comforted by having Alice as a professional legacy.

So it's OK that I won't set foot in the Promised Land. It's still a wonderful sight.

V

IT'S ABOUT
HOW TO LIVE
YOUR LIFE

This section may be called "It's About How to Live Your Life," but it's really about how I've tried to live mine. I guess it's my way of saying: Here's what worked for me.

—R.P.

28

Dream Big

MEN FIRST walked on the moon during the summer of 1969, when I was eight years old. I knew then that pretty much anything was possible. It was as if all of us, all over the world, had been given permission to dream big dreams.

I was at camp that summer, and after the lunar module landed, all of us were brought to the main farm house, where a television was set up. The astronauts were taking a long time getting organized before they could climb down the ladder and walk on the lunar surface. I understood. They had a lot of gear, a lot of details to attend to. I was patient.

But the people running the camp kept looking at their watches. It was already after eleven. Eventually, while smart decisions were being made on the moon, a dumb one was made here on Earth. It had gotten too late. All of us kids were sent back to our tents to go to sleep.

I was completely peeved at the camp directors. The thought

in my head was this: "My species has gotten off of our planet and landed in a new world for the first time, and you people think bedtime matters?"

But when I got home a few weeks later, I learned that my dad had taken a photo of our TV set the second Neil Armstrong set foot on the moon. He had preserved the moment for me, knowing it could help trigger big dreams. We still have that photo in a scrapbook.

I understand the arguments about how the billions of dollars spent to put men on the moon could have been used to fight poverty and hunger on Earth. But, look, I'm a scientist who sees inspiration as the ultimate tool for doing good.

When you use money to fight poverty, it can be of great value, but too often, you're working at the margins. When you're putting people on the moon, you're inspiring all of us

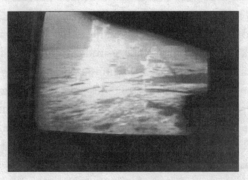

The moon landing on our television, courtesy of my father.

to achieve the maximum of human potential, which is how our greatest problems will eventually be solved.

Give yourself permission to dream. Fuel your kids' dreams, too. Once in a while, that might even mean letting them stay up past their bedtimes.

29

Earnest Is Better Than Hip

I'LL TAKE an earnest person over a hip person every time, because hip is short-term. Earnest is long-term.

Earnestness is highly underestimated. It comes from the core, while hip is trying to impress you with the surface.

"Hip" people love parodies. But there's no such thing as a timeless parody, is there? I have more respect for the earnest guy who does something that can last for generations, and that hip people feel the *need* to parody.

When I think of someone who is earnest, I think of a Boy Scout who works hard and becomes an Eagle Scout. When I was interviewing people to work for me, and I came upon a candidate who had been an Eagle Scout, I'd almost always try to hire him. I knew there had to be an earnestness about him that outweighed any superficial urges toward hipness.

Think about it. Becoming an Eagle Scout is just about the only thing you can put on your resume at age fifty that you

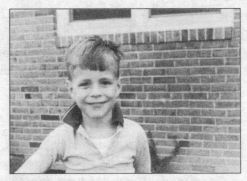

My wardrobe hasn't changed.

did at age fourteen—and it still impresses. (Despite my efforts at earnestness, I never did make it to Eagle Scout.)

Fashion, by the way, is commerce masquerading as hip. I'm not at all interested in fashion, which is why I rarely buy new clothes. The fact that fashion goes out of fashion and then comes back into fashion based solely on what a few people somewhere think they can sell, well to me, that's insanity.

My parents taught me: You buy new clothes when your old clothes wear out. Anyone who saw what I wore to my last lecture knows this is advice I live by!

My wardrobe is far from hip. It's kind of earnest. It's going to carry me through just fine.

30

Raising the White Flag

My mother always calls me "Randolph."

She was raised on a small dairy farm in Virginia during the Depression, wondering if there'd be enough food for dinner. She picked "Randolph" because it felt like the name some classy Virginian might have. And that may be why I rejected it and abhorred it. Who wants a name like that?

And yet my mother kept at it. As a teen, I confronted her. "Do you really believe your right to name me supersedes my right to have my own identity?"

"Yes, Randolph, I do," she said.

Well, at least we knew where we stood!

By the time I got to college, I had had enough. She'd send me mail addressed to "Randolph Pausch." I'd scrawl "no such person at this address" on the envelope, and send the letters back unopened.

In a great act of compromise, my mom began addressing letters to "R. Pausch." Those, I'd open. But then, when we'd talk on the phone, she'd revert back to old form. "Randolph, did you get our letter?"

Now, all these years later, I've given up. I am so appreciative of my mother on so many fronts that if she wants to burden me with an unnecessary "olph" whenever she's around, I'm more than happy put up with it. Life's too short.

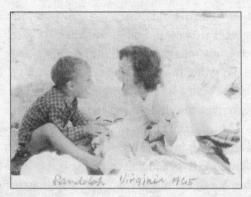

Randolph Virginia 1945

Mom and me, at the beach.

Somehow, with the passage of time, and the deadlines that life imposes, surrendering became the right thing to do.

31

Let's Make a Deal

WHEN I was in grad school, I developed the habit of tipping back in my chair at the dining-room table. I would do it whenever I visited my parents' house, and my mother would constantly reprimand me. "Randolph, you are going to break that chair!" she'd say.

I liked leaning back in the chair. It felt comfortable. And

the chair seemed to handle itself on two legs just fine. So, meal after meal after meal, I'd lean back and she'd reprimand.

One day, my mother said, "Stop leaning back in that chair. I'm not going to tell you again!"

Now *that* sounded like something I could sign up for. So I suggested we create a contract—a parent/child agreement in writing. If I broke the chair, I'd have to pay to replace not *just* the chair . . . but, as an added inducement, the entire dining-room set. (Replacing an individual chair on a twenty-year-old set would be impossible.) But, until I actually broke the chair, no lectures from Mom.

Certainly my mother was right; I was putting stress on the chair legs. But both of us decided that this agreement was a way to avoid arguments. I was acknowledging my responsibility in case there was damage. She was in the position of being able to say "You should always listen to your mother" if one of the chair legs cracked.

The chair has never broken. And whenever I visit her house and lean backward, the agreement still stands. There's not a cross word. In fact, the whole dynamic has changed. I won't say Mom has gone as far as to actually *encourage* me to lean back. But I do think she has long had her eye on a new dining-room set.

32
Don't Complain, Just Work Harder

TOO MANY people go through life complaining about their problems. I've always believed that if you took one-tenth the energy you put into complaining and applied it to solving the problem, you'd be surprised by how well things can work out.

I've known some terrific non-complainers in my life. One was Sandy Blatt, my landlord during graduate school. When he was a young man, a truck backed into him while he was unloading boxes into the cellar of a building. He toppled backwards down the steps and into the cellar. "How far was the fall?" I asked. His answer was simple: "Far enough." He spent the rest of his life as a quadriplegic.

Sandy had been a phenomenal athlete, and at the time of the accident, he was engaged to be married. He didn't want to be a burden to his fiancée so he told her, "You didn't sign on for this. I'll understand if you want to back out. You can go in peace." And she did.

I met Sandy when he was in his thirties, and he just wowed me with his attitude. He had this incredible non-whining aura about him. He had worked hard and become a licensed marriage counselor. He got married and adopted children. And when he talked about his medical issues, he did so matter-of-factly. He once explained to me that temperature changes were hard on quadriplegics because they can't shiver. "Pass me that blanket, will you, Randy?" he'd say. And that was it.

My favorite non-complainer of all time may be Jackie Robinson, the first African American to play Major League Baseball. He endured racism that many young people today couldn't even fathom. He knew he had to play better than the white guys, and he knew he had to work harder. So that's what he did. He vowed not to complain, even if fans spit on him.

I used to have a photo of Jackie Robinson hanging in my office, and it saddened me that so many students couldn't identify him, or knew little about him. Many never even noticed the photo. Young people raised on color TV don't spend a lot of time looking at black-and-white images.

That's too bad. There are no better role models than people like Jackie Robinson and Sandy Blatt. The message in their stories is this: Complaining does not work as a strategy. We all have finite time and energy. Any time we spend whining is unlikely to help us achieve our goals. And it won't make us happier.

33

Treat the Disease, Not the Symptom

YEARS AGO, I dated a lovely young woman who was a few thousand dollars in debt. She was completely stressed out about this. Every month, more interest would be added to her debts.

To deal with her stress, she would go every Tuesday night to a meditation and yoga class. This was her one free night, and she said it seemed to be helping her. She would breathe in, imagining that she was finding ways to deal with her debts. She would breathe out, telling herself that her money problems would one day be behind her.

It went on like this, Tuesday after Tuesday.

Finally, one day I looked through her finances with her. I figured out that if she spent four or five months working a part-time job on Tuesday nights, she could actually pay off all the money she owed.

I told her I had nothing against yoga or meditation. But I did think it's always best to try to treat the disease first. Her symptoms were stress and anxiety. Her disease was the money she owed.

"Why don't you get a job on Tuesday nights and skip yoga for a while?" I suggested.

This was something of a revelation to her. And she took my advice. She became a Tuesday-night waitress and soon enough paid off her debts. After that, she could go back to yoga and really breathe easier.

34

Don't Obsess Over What People Think

I'VE FOUND that a substantial fraction of many people's days is spent worrying about what others think of them. If nobody ever worried about what was in other people's heads, we'd all be 33 percent more effective in our lives and on our jobs.

How did I come up with 33 percent? I'm a scientist. I like exact numbers, even if I can't always prove them. So let's just run with 33 percent.

I used to tell anyone who worked in my research group: "You don't ever have to worry about what I'm thinking. Good or bad, I'll let you know what's in my head."

That meant when I wasn't happy about something, I spoke up, often directly and not always tactfully. But on the positive side, I was able to reassure people: "If I haven't said anything, you have nothing to worry about."

Students and colleagues came to appreciate that, and they didn't waste a lot of time obsessing over "What is Randy thinking?" Because mostly, what I was thinking was this: I have people on my team who are 33 percent more effective than everyone else. That's what was in my head.

35

Start By Sitting Together

W HEN I have to work with other people, I try to imagine us sitting together with a deck of cards. My impulse is always to put all my cards on the table, face up, and to say to the group, "OK, what can we collectively make of this hand?"

Being able to work well in a group is a vital and necessary skill in both the work world and in families. As a way to teach this, I'd always put my students into teams to work on projects.

Over the years, improving group dynamics became a bit of an obsession for me. On the first day of each semester, I'd break my class into about a dozen four-person groups. Then, on the second day of class, I'd give them a one-page handout I'd written titled "Tips for Working Successfully in a Group." We'd go over it, line by line. Some students found my tips to be beneath them. They rolled their eyes. They assumed they knew how to play well with others: They had learned it in kindergarten. They didn't need my rudimentary little pointers.

But the most self-aware students embraced the advice. They sensed that I was trying to teach them the fundamentals. It was a little like Coach Graham coming to practice without a football. Among my tips:

Meet people properly: It all starts with the introduction. Exchange contact information. Make sure you can pronounce everyone's names.

Find things you have in common: You can almost always find something in common with another person, and from there, it's much easier to address issues where you have differences. Sports cut across boundaries of race and wealth. And if nothing else, we all have the weather in common.

Try for optimal meeting conditions: Make sure no one is hungry, cold or tired. Meet over a meal if you can; food *softens* a meeting. That's why they "do lunch" in Hollywood.

Let everyone talk: Don't finish someone's sentences. And talking louder or faster doesn't make your idea any better.

Check egos at the door: When you discuss ideas, label them and write them down. The label should be descriptive of the idea, not the originator: "the bridge story" not "Jane's story."

Praise each other: Find something nice to say, even if it's a stretch. The worst ideas can have silver linings if you look hard enough.

Phrase alternatives as questions: Instead of "I think we should do A, not B," try "What if we did A, instead of B?" That allows people to offer comments rather than defend one choice.

At the end of my little lesson, I told my students I'd found a good way to take attendance. "It's easier for me if I just call you by group," I'd say. "Group One raise your hands . . . Group Two? . . ."

As I called off each group, hands would go up. "Did anybody notice anything about this?" I'd ask. No one had an answer. So I'd call off the groups again. "Group One? . . .

Group Two? . . . Group Three? . . ." All around the room, hands shot up again.

Sometimes, you have to resort to cheesy theatrics to break through to students, especially on issues where they think they know everything. So here's what I did:

I kept going with my attendance drill until finally my voice was raised. "Why on earth are all of you still sitting with your friends?" I'd ask. "Why aren't you sitting with the people in your group?"

Some knew my irritation was for effect, but everyone took me seriously. "I'm going to walk out of this room," I said, "and I'll be back in sixty seconds. When I return, I expect you to be sitting with your groups! Does everyone understand?" I'd waltz out and I'd hear the panic in the room, as students gathered up their book bags and reshuffled themselves into groups.

When I returned, I explained that my tips for working in groups were not meant to insult their intelligence or maturity. I just wanted to show them that they had missed something simple—the fact that they needed to sit with their partners—and so they could certainly benefit from reviewing the rest of the basics.

At the next class, and for the rest of the semester, my students (no dummies), always sat with their groups.

36

Look for the Best in Everybody

THIS IS beautiful advice that I got once from Jon Snoddy, my hero at Disney Imagineering. I just was so taken with the way he put it. "If you wait long enough," he said, "people will surprise and impress you."

As he saw things: When you're frustrated with people, when they've made you angry, it just may be because you haven't given them enough time.

Jon warned me that sometimes this took great patience—even years. "But in the end," he said, "people will show you their good side. Almost everybody has a good side. Just keep waiting. It will come out."

37

Watch What They Do, Not What They Say

MY DAUGHTER is just eighteen months, so I can't tell her this now, but when she's old enough, I want Chloe to know something a female colleague once told me, which is good advice for young ladies everywhere. In fact, pound for pound, it's the best advice I've ever heard.

My colleague told me: "It took a long time, but I've finally figured it out. When it comes to men who are romantically interested in you, it's really simple. Just ignore everything they say and only pay attention to what they do."

That's it. So here it is, for Chloe.

And as I think about it, some day it could come in pretty useful for Dylan and Logan, too.

38

If at First You Don't Succeed . . .

... TRY, TRY a cliché.

I love clichés. A lot of them, anyway. I have great respect for the old chestnuts. As I see it, the reason clichés are repeated so often is because they're so often right on the money.

Educators shouldn't be afraid of clichés. You know why? Because kids don't know most of them! They're a new audience, and they're inspired by clichés. I've seen it again and again in my classroom.

Dance with the one who brung you. That's a cliché my parents always told me, and it applies far beyond prom night. It should be a mantra in the business world, in academia, and at home. It's a reminder about loyalty and appreciation.

Luck is what happens when preparation meets opportunity. That comes from Seneca, the Roman philosopher who was born in 5 B.C. It'll be worth repeating for another two thousand years, at least.

Whether you think you can or can't, you're right. That is from my cliché repertoire for incoming students.

Other than that, Mrs. Lincoln, how was the play? I'd say that to students as a reminder not to focus on little issues, while ignoring the major ones.

I love a lot of pop culture clichés, too. I don't mind when my children watch *Superman,* not because he's strong and can fly, but because he fights for "truth, justice and the American way." I *love* that line.

I love the movie *Rocky.* I even love the theme music. And what I liked most about the original *Rocky* movie was that Rocky didn't care if he won the fight that ends the film. He just didn't want to get knocked out. That was his goal. During the most painful times of my treatment, Rocky was an inspiration because he reminded me: It's not how hard you hit. It's how hard you get hit . . . and keep moving forward.

Of course, of all the clichés in the world, I love football clichés the most. Colleagues were used to the sight of me wandering the halls of Carnegie Mellon tossing a football up and down in front of me. It helped me think. They'd probably say I thought football metaphors had the same effect. But some of my students, female and male, had trouble adjusting. They'd be discussing computer algorithms and I'd be speaking football. "Sorry," I'd tell them. "But it will be easier for you to learn the basics of football than for me to learn a new set of life clichés."

I liked my students to win one for the Gipper, to go out and execute, to keep the drive alive, to march down the field, to avoid costly turnovers and to win games in the trenches even if they were gonna feel it on Monday. My students knew: It's not just whether you win or lose, it's how you play the cliché.

39

Be the First Penguin

EXPERIENCE IS what you get when you didn't get what you wanted.

That's an expression I learned when I took a sabbatical at Electronic Arts, the video-game maker. It just stuck with me, and I've ended up repeating it again and again to students.

It's a phrase worth considering at every brick wall we encounter, and at every disappointment. It's also a reminder that failure is not just acceptable, it's often essential.

When I taught the "Building Virtual Worlds" course, I encouraged students to attempt hard things and to not worry about failing. I wanted to reward that way of thinking. So at the end of each semester, I'd present one team of students with a stuffed animal—a penguin. It was called "The First Penguin Award" and went to the team that took the biggest gamble in trying new ideas or new technology, while failing to achieve their stated goals. In essence, it was an award for "glorious failure," and it celebrated out-of-the-box thinking and using imagination in a daring way.

The other students came to understand: "First Penguin" winners were losers who were definitely going somewhere.

The title of the award came from the notion that when penguins are about to jump into water that might contain predators, well, somebody's got to be the first penguin. I originally called it "The Best Failure Award," but failure has so many negative connotations that students couldn't get past the word itself.

Over the years, I also made a point of telling my students that in the entertainment industry, there are countless failed products. It's not like building houses, where every house built can be lived in by someone. A video game can be created and never make it through research and development. Or else it comes out and no one wants to play it. Yes, video-game creators who've had successes are greatly valued. But those who've had failures are valued, too—sometimes even more so.

Start-up companies often prefer to hire a chief executive with a failed start-up in his or her background. The person who failed often knows how to avoid future failures. The person who knows only success can be more oblivious to all the pitfalls.

Experience is what you get when you didn't get what you wanted. And experience is often the most valuable thing you have to offer.

40

Get People's Attention

———————

So MANY of my students were incredibly smart. I knew they would get into the working world and create terrific new software programs, animation projects and entertainment devices. I also knew they had the potential to frustrate millions of people in the process.

Those of us who are engineers and computer scientists don't always think about how to build things so they're easy to use. A lot of us are terrible at explaining complex tasks in simple ways. Ever read the instruction booklet for a VCR? Then you've lived the frustration I'm talking about.

That's why I wanted to impress upon my students the importance of thinking about the end users of their creations. How could I make clear to them how important it was not to create technology that is frustrating? I came up with a surefire attention-getter.

When I taught a "user interface" class at the University of Virginia, I'd bring in a working VCR on the first day. I would put it on a desk in the front of the room. I would pull out a sledgehammer. I would destroy the VCR.

Then I would say: "When we make something hard to use, people get upset. They become so angry that they want to destroy it. We don't want to create things that people will want to destroy."

The students would look at me and I could tell they were shocked, bewildered and slightly amused. It was exciting for them. They were thinking: "I don't know who this guy is, but I'm definitely coming to class tomorrow to check out his next stunt."

I sure got their attention. That's always the first step to solving an ignored problem. (When I left the University of Virginia for Carnegie Mellon, my friend and fellow professor Gabe Robins gave me a sledgehammer with a plaque attached. It read: "So many VCRs, so little time!")

All of the students from my days at UVa. are in the workforce now. As they go about creating new technologies, I hope that once in a while I come into their minds, swinging that sledgehammer, reminding them of the frustrated masses, yearning for simplicity.

41

The Lost Art of Thank-You Notes

S HOWING GRATITUDE is one of the simplest yet most powerful things humans can do for each other. And despite my love of efficiency, I think that thank-you notes are best done the old-fashioned way, with pen and paper.

Job interviewers and admissions officers see lots of applicants. They read tons of resumes from "A" students with many accomplishments. But they do not see many handwritten thank-you notes.

If you are a B+ student, your handwritten thank-you note will raise you at least a half-grade in the eyes of a future boss or admissions officer. You will become an "A" to them. And because handwritten notes have gotten so rare, they will remember you.

When I'd give this advice to my students, it was not to make them into calculating schemers, although I know some embraced it on those terms. My advice was more about helping them recognize that there are respectful, considerate things that can be done in life that will be appreciated by the recipient, and that only good things can result.

For instance, there was a young lady who applied to get into the ETC and we were about to turn her down. She had big dreams; she wanted to be a Disney Imagineer. Her grades, her exams and her portfolio were good, but not quite good enough, given how selective the ETC could afford to be. Before we put her into the "no" pile, I decided to page through her file one more time. As I did, I noticed a handwritten thank-you note had been slipped between the other pages.

The note hadn't been sent to me, my co-director Don Marinelli, or any other faculty member. Instead, she had mailed it to a non-faculty support staffer who had helped her with arrangements when she came to visit. This staff member held no sway over her application, so this was not a suck-up note. It was just a few words of thanks to somebody who, unbeknownst to her, happened to toss her note to him into her application folder. Weeks later, I came upon it.

Having unexpectedly caught her thanking someone just because it was the nice thing to do, I paused to reflect on this. She had written her note by hand. I liked that. "This tells me more than anything else in her file," I said to Don. I read through her materials again. I thought about her. Impressed by her note, I decided she was worth taking a chance on, and Don agreed.

She came to the ETC, got her master's degree, and is now a Disney Imagineer.

I've told her this story, and now she tells it to others.

Despite all that is now going on in my life and with my medical care, I still try to handwrite notes when it's important to do so. It's just the nice thing to do. And you never know what magic might happen after it arrives in someone's mailbox.

42

Loyalty Is a Two-Way Street

WHEN DENNIS Cosgrove was an undergraduate student of mine at the University of Virginia in the early 1990s, I found him to be impressive. He was doing terrific work in my computer lab. He was a teaching assistant in the operating systems course. He was taking graduate level courses. And he was an A student.

Well, in most classes he was an A student. In Calculus III, he was an F student. It wasn't that he lacked the ability. He was just so focused on his computer courses, being a teaching assistant, and a research assistant in my lab that he simply stopped going to calculus class.

That turned out to be a serious problem, as it was not the first time he had a semester in which he earned straight A's with an F.

It was two weeks into a new semester when Dennis's checkered academic record caught the attention of a certain dean. He knew how smart Dennis was; he had seen his SAT and AP scores. In his view, the F's were all due to attitude, not aptitude. He wanted to expel Dennis. But I knew Dennis had never received a single warning about any of this. In fact, all of his A's offset his F's to the point where he couldn't even be academically suspended. Yet, the Dean invoked an obscure rule that left expulsion on the table. I decided to go to bat for my student. "Look," I told the dean, "Dennis is a strong rocket with no fins. He's been a star in my lab. If we kick him out right now, we'll be missing the whole point of what we're here for. We're here to teach, to nurture. I know Dennis is going somewhere special. We can't just dump him."

The dean was not happy with me. In his view, I was a young professor getting pushy.

Then I got even pushier. I went tactical. The new semester had already begun. The university had cashed Dennis's tuition check. By doing so, as I saw it, we were telling him he was welcome to remain as a student. Had we expelled him before the semester, he could have tried to enroll in another school. Now it was too late for that.

I asked the dean: "What if he hires a lawyer to argue this? I might just testify on his behalf. Do you want one of your faculty members testifying against the university?"

The dean was taken aback. "You're a junior faculty member," he said. "You're not even tenured yet. Why are you sticking your neck out and making this the battle you want to undertake?"

"I'll tell you the reason," I said. "I want to vouch for Dennis because I believe in him."

The dean took a long look at me. "I'm going to remember this when your tenure case comes up," he said. In other words, if Dennis screwed up again, my judgment would be seriously questioned.

"That's a deal," I told the dean. And Dennis was able to stay in school.

He passed Calculus III, did us all proud, and after graduating, went on to become an award-winning star in computer science. He's been part of my life and my labs ever since. In fact, he was one of the early fathers of the Alice project. As a designer, he did groundbreaking programming work to help make the virtual reality system more accessible to young people.

I went to bat for Dennis when he was twenty-one years old. Now at age thirty-seven, he is going to go to bat for me. I've entrusted him with carrying Alice into the future as the research scientist designing and implementing my professional legacy.

I enabled Dennis's dream way back when he needed it . . . and now that I need it, he is enabling mine.

43

The Friday Night Solution

I GOT TENURE a year earlier than people usually do. That seemed to impress other junior faculty members.

"Wow, you got tenure early," they'd say to me. "What was your secret?"

I said, "It's pretty simple. Call me any Friday night in my office at ten o'clock and I'll tell you." (Of course, this was before I had a family.)

A lot of people want a shortcut. I find the best shortcut is the long way, which is basically two words: work hard.

As I see it, if you work more hours than somebody else, during those hours you learn more about your craft. That can make you more efficient, more able, even happier. Hard work is like compounded interest in the bank. The rewards build faster.

The same is true in your life outside of your job. All my adult life I've felt drawn to ask long-married couples how they were able to stay together. All of them said the same thing: "We worked hard at it."

44

Show Gratitude

Not long after I got tenure at the University of Virginia, I took my entire fifteen-person research team down to Disney World for a week as my way of saying thank you.

A fellow professor took me aside and said, "Randy, how could you do that?" Perhaps he thought I was setting a precedent that other soon-to-be-tenured professors would be unwilling to equal.

"How could I do that?" I answered. "These people just worked their butts off and got me the best job in the world for life. How could I *not* do that?"

So the sixteen of us headed down to Florida in a large van. We had a complete blast, and I made sure we all got some education with our entertainment, too. Along the way, we stopped at various universities and visited computer research groups.

The Disney trip was gratitude easily delivered. It was a tangible gift, and it was perfect because it was an experience I could share with people I cared about.

Not everyone is so easily thanked, however.

One of my greatest mentors was Andy van Dam, my computer science professor when I was at Brown. He gave me wise counsel. He changed my life. I could never adequately pay him back, so I just have to pay it forward.

I always liked telling my students: "Go out and do for others what somebody did for you." Riding down to Disney World, talking to my students about their dreams and goals, I was trying my best to do just that.

45

Send Out Thin Mints

As part of my responsibilities, I used to be an academic reviewer. That meant I'd have to ask other professors to read densely written research papers and review them. It could be tedious, sleep-inducing work. So I came up with an idea. I'd send a box of Girl Scout Thin Mints with every paper that needed to be reviewed. "Thank you for agreeing to do this," I'd write. "The enclosed Thin Mints are your reward. But no fair eating them until you review the paper."

That put a smile on people's faces. And I never had to call and nag them. They had the box of Thin Mints on their desks. They knew what they had to do.

Sure, sometimes I had to send a reminder email. But when I'd ping people, all I needed was one sentence: "Did you eat the Thin Mints yet?"

I've found Thin Mints are a great communication tool. They're also a sweet reward for a job well done.

46

All You Have Is What You Bring With You

─────────

I'VE ALWAYS felt a need to be prepared for whatever situation I've found myself in. When I leave the house, what do I need to bring? When I teach a class, what questions should I anticipate? When I'm preparing for my family's future without me, what documents should I have in place?

My mother recalls taking me to a grocery store when I was seven years old. She and I got to the checkout counter, and she realized she'd forgotten a couple of items on her shopping list. She left me with the cart and she ran off to get what she needed.

"I'll be right back," she said.

She was gone just a few minutes, but in that time, I had loaded all the items on the belt and everything was rung up. I was left staring at the cashier, who was staring at me. The cashier decided to make sport of the situation. "Do you have money for me, son?" she said. "I'll need to be paid."

I didn't realize she was just trying to amuse herself. So I stood there, mortified and embarrassed.

By the time my mom returned, I was angry. "You left me here with no money! This lady asked me for the money, and I had nothing to give her!"

Now that I'm an adult, you'll never catch me with less

than $200 in my wallet. I want to be prepared in case I need it. Sure, I could lose my wallet or it could be stolen. But for a guy making a reasonable living, $200 is an amount worth risking. By contrast, not having cash on hand when you need it is potentially a much bigger problem.

I've always admired people who are over-prepared. In college, I had a classmate named Norman Meyrowitz. One day he was giving a presentation on an overhead projector and in the middle of his talk, the lightbulb on the projector blew out. There was an audible groan from the audience. We'd have to wait ten minutes until someone found a new projector.

"It's okay," Norm announced. "There's nothing to worry about."

We watched him walk over to his knapsack and pull something out. He had brought along a spare bulb for the overhead projector. Who would even think of that?

Our professor, Andy van Dam, happened to be sitting next to me. He leaned over and said, "This guy is going places." He had that right. Norm became a top executive at Macromedia Inc., where his efforts have affected almost everyone who uses the Internet today.

Another way to be prepared is to think negatively.

Yes, I'm a great optimist. But when trying to make a decision, I often think of the worst-case scenario. I call it "The Eaten By Wolves Factor." If I do something, what's the most terrible thing that could happen? Would I be eaten by wolves?

One thing that makes it possible to be an optimist is if

you have a contingency plan for when all hell breaks loose. There are a lot of things I don't worry about because I have a plan in place if they do.

I've often told my students: "When you go into the wilderness, the only thing you can count on is what you take with you." And essentially, the wilderness is anywhere but your home or office. So take money. Bring your repair kit. Imagine the wolves. Pack a lightbulb. Be prepared.

47

A Bad Apology Is Worse Than No Apology

APOLOGIES ARE not pass/fail. I always told my students: When giving an apology, any performance lower than an A really doesn't cut it.

Halfhearted or insincere apologies are often worse than not apologizing at all because recipients find them insulting. If you've done something wrong in your dealings with another person, it's as if there's an infection in your relationship. A good apology is like an antibiotic; a bad apology is like rubbing salt in the wound.

Working in groups was crucial in my classes, and friction between students was unavoidable. Some students wouldn't pull their load. Others were so full of themselves that they'd belittle their partners. By mid-semester, apologies were *always* in order. When students wouldn't do it, everything would spin out of control. So I'd often give classes my little routine about apologies.

I'd start by describing the two classic bad apologies:

1) "I'm sorry you feel hurt by what I've done." (This is an attempt at an emotional salve, but it's obvious you don't want to put any medicine in the wound.)
2) "I apologize for what I did, but you also need to apologize to me for what you've done." (That's not giving an apology. That's asking for one.)

Proper apologies have three parts:

1) What I did was wrong.
2) I feel badly that I hurt you.
3) How do I make this better?

Yes, some people may take advantage of you when answering question three. But most people will be genuinely appreciative of your make-good efforts. They may tell you how to make it better in some small, easy way. And often, they'll work harder to help make things better themselves.

Students would say to me: "What if I apologize and the other person doesn't apologize back?" I'd tell them: "That's not something you can control, so don't let it eat at you."

If other people owe you an apology, and your words of apology to them are proper and heartfelt, you still may not hear from them for a while. After all, what are the odds that they get to the right emotional place to apologize at the exact moment you do? So just be patient. Many times in my career, I saw students apologize, and then several days later, their teammates came around. Your patience will be both appreciated and rewarded.

48

Tell the Truth

IF I could only give three words of advice, they would be "tell the truth." If I got three more words, I'd add: "All the time." My parents taught me that "you're only as good as your word," and there's no better way to say it.

Honesty is not only morally right, it's also efficient. In a culture where everyone tells the truth, you can save a lot of time double-checking. When I taught at the University of Virginia, I *loved* the honor code. If a student was sick and needed a makeup exam, I didn't need to create a new one. The student just "pledged" that he hadn't talked to anybody about the exam, and I gave the old one.

People lie for lots of reasons, often because it seems like a way to get what they want with less effort. But like many short-term strategies, it's ineffective long-term. You run into people again later, and they remember you lied to them. And they tell lots of other people about it. That's what amazes me about lying. Most people who have told a lie think they got away with it . . . when in fact, they didn't.

49

Get in Touch with Your Crayon Box

P EOPLE WHO know me sometimes complain that I see things in black or white.

In fact, one of my colleagues would tell people: "Go to Randy if you want black-and-white advice. But if you want gray advice, he's not the guy."

OK. I stand guilty as charged, especially when I was younger. I used to say that my crayon box had only two colors in it: black and white. I guess that's why I love computer science, because most everything is true or false.

As I've gotten older, though, I've learned to appreciate that a good crayon box might have more than two colors. But I still think that if you run your life the right way, you'll wear out the black and the white before the more nuanced colors.

In any case, whatever the color, I love crayons.

At my last lecture, I had brought along several hundred of them. I wanted everyone to get one when they walked into the lecture hall, but in the confusion, I forgot to have the folks at the door pass them out. Too bad. My plan was this: As I spoke about childhood dreams, I'd ask everyone to close their eyes and rub their crayons in their fingers—to feel the texture, the paper, the wax. Then I'd have them bring their crayons up to their noses and take a good long whiff. Smelling a crayon takes you right back to childhood, doesn't it?

I once saw a colleague do a similar crayon routine with a group of people, and it had inspired me. In fact, since then, I've often carried a crayon in my shirt pocket. When I need to go back in time, I put it under my nose and I take another hit.

I'm partial to the black crayon and the white crayon, but that's just me. Any color has the same potency. Breathe it in. You'll see.

50

The $100,000 Salt and Pepper Shaker

WHEN I was twelve years old and my sister was fourteen, our family went to Disney World in Orlando. Our parents figured we were just old enough to roam a bit around the park without being monitored. In those days before cell phones, Mom and Dad told us to be careful, picked a spot where we would meet ninety minutes later, and then they let us take off.

Think of the thrill that was! We were in the coolest place imaginable and we had the freedom to explore it on our own. We were also extremely grateful to our parents for taking us there, and for recognizing we were mature enough to be by ourselves. So we decided to thank them by pooling our allowances and getting them a present.

We went into a store and found what we considered the perfect gift: a ceramic salt and pepper shaker featuring two bears hanging off a tree, each one holding a shaker. We paid ten dollars for the gift, headed out of the store, and skipped up Main Street in search of the next attraction.

I was holding the gift, and in a horrible instant, it slipped out of my hands. The thing broke on impact. My sister and I were both in tears.

An adult guest in the park saw what happened and came over to us. "Take it back to the store," she suggested. "I'm sure they'll give you a new one."

"I can't do that," I said. "It was my fault. I dropped it. Why would the store give us another one?"

"Try anyway," the adult said. "You never know."

So we went back to the store . . . and we didn't lie. We explained what happened. The employees in the store listened to our sad story, smiled at us . . . and told us we could have a new salt and pepper shaker. They even said it was *their* fault because they hadn't wrapped the original salt and pepper shaker well enough! Their message was, "Our packaging should have been able to withstand a fall due to a twelve-year-old's overexcitement."

I was in shock. Not just gratitude, but disbelief. My sister and I left the store completely giddy.

When my parents learned of the incident, it *really* increased their appreciation of Disney World. In fact, that one customer-service decision over a ten-dollar salt and pepper shaker would end up earning Disney more than $100,000.

Let me explain.

Years later, as a Disney Imagineering consultant, I would sometimes end up chatting with executives pretty high up the Disney chain of command, and wherever I could I would tell them the story of the salt and pepper shaker.

I would explain how the people in that gift shop made my sister and me feel so good about Disney, and how that led my parents to appreciate the institution on a whole other level.

My parents made visits to Disney World an integral part of their volunteer work. They had a twenty-two-passenger bus they would use to drive English-as-a-second-language students from Maryland down to see the park. For more than twenty years, my dad bought tickets for dozens of kids to go to Disney World. I went on most of those trips.

All in all, since that day, my family has spent more than $100,000 at Disney World on tickets, food and souvenirs for ourselves and others.

When I tell this story to today's Disney executives, I always end it by asking them: "If I sent a child into one of your stores with a broken salt and pepper shaker today, would your policies allow your workers to be kind enough to replace it?"

The executives squirm at the question. They know the answer: Probably not.

That's because nowhere in their accounting system are they able to measure how a ten-dollar salt and pepper shaker might yield $100,000. And so it's easy to envision that a child today would be out of luck, sent out of a store with empty hands.

My message is this: There is more than one way to measure profits and losses. On every level, institutions can and should have a heart.

My mom still has that $100,000 salt and pepper shaker. The day the folks at Disney World replaced it was a great day for us . . . and not a bad one for Disney!

51

No Job Is Beneath You

IT'S BEEN well-documented that there is a growing sense of entitlement among young people today. I have certainly seen that in my classrooms.

So many graduating seniors have this notion that they should be hired because of their creative brilliance. Too many are unhappy with the idea of starting at the bottom.

My advice has always been: "You ought to be thrilled you

got a job in the mailroom. And when you get there, here's what you do: Be really great at sorting mail."

No one wants to hear someone say: "I'm not good at sorting mail because the job is beneath me." No job should be beneath us. And if you can't (or won't) sort mail, where is the proof that you can do anything?

After our ETC students were hired by companies for internships or first jobs, we'd often ask the firms to give us feedback on how they were doing. Their bosses almost never had anything negative to say about their abilities or their technical chops. But when we did get negative feedback, it was almost always about how the new employees were too big for their britches. Or that they were already eyeing the corner offices.

When I was fifteen, I worked at an orchard hoeing strawberries, and most of my coworkers were day laborers. A couple of teachers worked there, too, earning a little extra cash for the summer. I made a comment to my dad about the job being beneath those teachers. (I guess I was implying that the job was beneath me, too.) My dad gave me the tongue-lashing of a lifetime. He believed manual labor was beneath no one. He said he'd prefer that I worked hard and became the best ditch-digger in the world rather than coasting along as a self-impressed elitist behind a desk.

I went back into that strawberry field and I still didn't like the job. But I had heard my dad's words. I watched my attitude and I hoed a little harder.

52

Know Where You Are

"OK, PROFESSOR Boy, what can you do for us?"

That was the greeting I received from Mk Haley, a twenty-seven-year-old Imagineer who was given the job of babysitting me during my sabbatical at Disney.

I had arrived in a place where my academic credentials meant nothing. I became a traveler in a foreign land who had to find a way to come up with the local currency—fast!

For years, I've told my students about this experience because it's a crucial lesson.

Although I had achieved my childhood dream of being an Imagineer, I had gone from being the top dog in my academic research lab to an odd duck in a rough-and-tumble pond. I had to figure out how my wonky ways could fit in this make-or-break creative culture.

I worked on the Aladdin virtual reality attraction then being tested at Epcot. I joined Imagineers interviewing guests about how they liked the ride. Did they get dizzy, disoriented, nauseated?

Some of my new colleagues complained that I was applying academic values that wouldn't work in the real world. They said I was too focused on poring over data, too insistent on approaching things scientifically rather than emotionally. It was hard-core academia (me) versus hard-core entertainment (them). Finally, though, after I figured out a way to save twenty seconds per guest by loading the ride differently, I gained some street cred with those Imagineers who had their doubts about me.

The reason I tell this story is to emphasize how sensitive you need to be when crossing from one culture to another—in my students' cases, from school to their first job.

As it turned out, at the end of my sabbatical, Imagineering offered me a full-time job. After much agonizing, I turned it down. The call of teaching was too strong. But because I'd figured out how to navigate in both academia and the entertainment industry, Disney found a way to keep me involved. I became a once-a-week consultant to Imagineering, which I did happily for ten years.

If you can find your footing between two cultures, sometimes you can have the best of both worlds.

53
Never Give Up

WHEN I was a senior in high school, I applied to Brown University and didn't get in. I was on the wait list. I called the admissions office until they eventually decided they might as well accept me. They saw how badly I wanted in. Tenacity got me over the brick wall.

When it was time to graduate from Brown, it never occurred to me in a million years to go to graduate school. People in my family got an education and then got jobs. They didn't keep getting an education.

But Andy van Dam, my "Dutch uncle" and mentor at Brown, advised me, "Get yourself a PhD. Be a professor."

"Why should I do that?" I asked him.

And he said: "Because you're such a good salesman, and if you go work for a company, they're going to use you as a salesman. If you're going to be a salesman, you might as well be selling something worthwhile, like education."

I am forever grateful for that advice.

Andy told me to apply to Carnegie Mellon, where he had sent a long string of his best students. "You'll get in, no problem," he said. He wrote me a letter of recommendation.

The Carnegie Mellon faculty read his glowing letter. They saw my reasonable grades and my lackluster graduate-exam scores. They reviewed my application.

And they rejected me.

I was accepted into other PhD programs, but Carnegie Mellon didn't want me. So I went into Andy's office and dropped the rejection letter on his desk. "I want you to know how much Carnegie Mellon values your recommendations," I said.

Within seconds of the letter hitting his desk, he picked up the phone. "I'll fix this. I'll get you in," he said.

But I stopped him. "I don't want to do it that way," I told him.

So we made a deal. I would check out the schools that

accepted me. If I didn't feel comfortable at any of them, I'd come back to him and we'd talk.

The other schools ended up being such a bad fit that I soon found myself returning to Andy. I told him I had decided to skip graduate school and get a job.

"No, no, no," he said. "You've got to get your PhD, and you've got to go to Carnegie Mellon."

He picked up the phone and called Nico Habermann, the head of Carnegie Mellon's computer science department, who also happened to be Dutch. They talked about me in Dutch for a while, and then Andy hung up and told me: "Be in his office at 8 a.m. tomorrow."

Nico was a presence: an old-school, European-style academic. It was clear our meeting was only happening as a favor to his friend Andy. He asked me why he should be reconsidering my application, given that the department had already evaluated me. Speaking carefully, I said, "Since the time that I was reviewed, I won a full fellowship from the Office of Naval Research." Nico replied gravely, "Having money isn't part of our admissions criteria; we fund our students out of research grants." And then he stared at me. More precisely, he stared *through* me.

There are a few key moments in anyone's life. A person is fortunate if he can tell in hindsight when they happened. I knew in the moment that I was in one. With all the deference my young, arrogant self could muster, I said "I'm sorry, I didn't mean to imply it was about the money. It's just that they only awarded fifteen of these fellowships nationwide, so

I thought it an honor that would be relevant, and I apologize if that was presumptuous of me."

It was the only answer I had, but it was the truth. Very, very slowly, Nico's frozen visage thawed and we talked for a few minutes more.

After meeting with several other faculty, I ended up being accepted by Carnegie Mellon, and I got my PhD. It was a brick wall surmounted with a huge boost from a mentor and some sincere groveling.

Until I got on stage at my last lecture, I had never told students or colleagues at Carnegie Mellon that I had been rejected when I applied there. What was I afraid of? That they'd all think I wasn't smart enough to be in their company? That they'd take me less seriously?

It's interesting, the secrets you decide to reveal at the end of your life.

I should have been telling that story for years, because the moral is: If you want something bad enough, never give up (and take a boost when offered).

Brick walls are there for a reason. And once you get over them—even if someone has practically had to throw you over—it can be helpful to others to tell them how you did it.

54
Be a Communitarian

WE'VE PLACED a lot of emphasis in this country on the idea of people's *rights*. That's how it should be, but it makes no sense to talk about rights without also talking about responsibilities.

Rights have to come from somewhere, and they come from the community. In return, all of us have a responsibility to the community. Some people call this the "communitarian" movement, but I call it common sense.

This idea has been lost on a lot of us, and in my twenty years as a professor, I've noticed more and more students just don't get it. The notion that rights come with responsibilities is, literally, a strange concept to them.

I'd ask students to sign an agreement at the start of each semester, outlining their responsibilities and rights. They had to agree to work constructively in groups, to attend certain meetings, to help their peers by giving honest feedback. In return, they had the right to be in the class and to have their work critiqued and displayed.

Some students balked at my agreement. I think it's because we as adults aren't always great role models about being communitarians. For example: We all believe we have a right to a jury trial. And yet many people go to great lengths to get out of jury duty.

So I wanted my students to know. Everyone has to contribute to the common good. To not do so can be described in one word: selfish.

My dad taught this to us by example, but he also looked for novel ways to teach it to others. He did something very clever when he was a Little League baseball commissioner.

He had been having trouble rounding up volunteer umpires. It was a thankless job, in part because every time you called a strike or a ball, some kid or parent was sure you got it wrong. There was also the issue of fear: You had to stand there while kids with little or no control flailed their bats and threw wild pitches at you.

Anyway, my dad came up with an idea. Instead of getting adults to volunteer, he had the players from the older-age divisions serve as umpires for the younger kids. He made it an honor to be selected as an ump.

Several things happened as a result of this.

The kids who became umpires understood how hard a job it was and hardly ever argued with umpires again. They also felt good that they were lending a hand to the kids in the younger divisions. Meanwhile, the younger kids saw older role models who had embraced volunteering.

My dad had created a new set of communitarians. He knew: When we're connected to others, we become better people.

55

All You Have to Do Is Ask

O N   M Y dad's last trip to Disney World, he and I were waiting for the monorail with Dylan, who was then four years old. Dylan had this urge to sit in the vehicle's cool-looking nose-cone, with the driver. My theme-park-loving father thought that would be a huge kick, too.

"Too bad they don't let regular people sit up there," he said.

"Hmmmm," I said. "Actually, Dad, having been an Imagiiner, I've learned that there's a trick to getting to sit up front. Do you want to see it?"

He said sure.

So I walked over to the smiling Disney monorail attendant and said: "Excuse me, could the three of us please sit in the front car?"

"Certainly, sir," the attendant said. He opened the gate and we took our seats beside the driver. It was one of the only times in my life I ever saw my dad completely flabbergasted. "I said there was a trick," I told him as we sped toward the Magic Kingdom. "I didn't say it was a *hard* trick."

Sometimes, all you have to do is ask.

I've always been fairly adept at asking for things. I'm proud of the time I got up my courage and contacted Fred Brooks Jr., one of the most highly regarded computer scientists in the world. After beginning his career at IBM in the

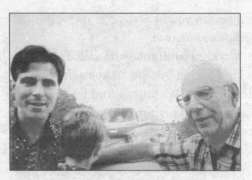

All we had to do was ask.

Fifties, he went on to found the computer science department at University of North Carolina. He is famous in our industry for saying, among other great things: "Adding manpower to a late software project makes it later." (This is now known as "Brooks Law.")

I was in my late twenties and still hadn't met the man, so I emailed him, asking: "If I drive down from Virginia to North Carolina, would it be possible to get thirty minutes of your time to talk?"

He responded: "If you drive all the way down here, I'll give you more than thirty minutes."

He gave me ninety minutes and became a lifelong mentor to me. Years later, he invited me to give a lecture at the University of North Carolina. That was the trip that led to the most seminal moment in my life—when I met Jai.

Sometimes, all you have to do is ask, and it can lead to all your dreams coming true.

These days, given my short road ahead, I've gotten even better at "just asking." As we all know, it often takes days to get medical results. Waiting around for medical news is not how I want to spend my time lately. So I always ask: "What's the fastest I can get these results?"

"Oh," they often respond. "We might be able to have it for you within an hour."

"*OK* then," I say . . . "I'm glad I asked!"

Ask those questions. Just ask them. More often than you'd suspect, the answer you'll get is, "Sure."

56

Make a Decision: Tigger or Eeyore

WHEN I told Carnegie Mellon's president, Jared Cohon, that I would be giving a last lecture, he said, "Please tell them about having fun, because that's what I will remember you for."

And I said, "I can do that, but it's kind of like a fish talking about the importance of water."

I mean, I don't know how *not* to have fun. I'm dying and I'm having fun. And I'm going to keep having fun every day I have left. Because there's no other way to play it.

I came to a realization about this very early in my life. As I see it, there's a decision we all have to make, and it seems perfectly captured in the Winnie-the-Pooh characters created by A. A. Milne. Each of us must decide: Am I a fun-loving Tigger or am I a sad-sack Eeyore? Pick a camp. I think it's clear where I stand on the great Tigger/Eeyore debate.

For my last Halloween, I had great fun. Jai and I dressed up as the Incredibles, and so did our three kids. I put a photo of us on my Web site letting everyone know what an "Incredible" family we were. The kids looked pretty super. I looked invincible with my fake cartoon muscles. I explained that chemo had not dramatically affected my superpowers, and I got tons of smiling emails in response.

I recently went on a short scuba-diving vacation with three of my best friends: my high school friend Jack Sheriff, my college roommate Scott Sherman, and my friend from Electronic Arts, Steve Seabolt. We all were aware of the subtext. These were my friends from various times in my life, and they were banding together to give me a farewell weekend.

My three friends didn't know each other well, but strong bonds formed quickly. All of us are grown men, but for much of the vacation it was as if we were thirteen years old. And we were all Tiggers.

We successfully avoided any emotional "I love you, man" dialogue related to my cancer. Instead, we just had fun. We reminisced, we horsed around and we made fun of each other. (Actually, it was mostly them making fun of *me* for the

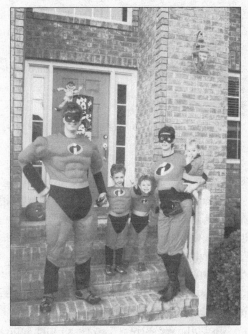

Chemo has not dramatically affected my superpowers.

"St. Randy of Pittsburgh" reputation I've gotten since my last
lecture. They know me, and they were having none of it.)

I won't let go of the Tigger inside me. I just can't see the
upside in becoming Eeyore. Someone asked me what I want
on my tombstone. I replied: "Randy Pausch: He Lived Thirty
Years After a Terminal Diagnosis."

I promise you. I could pack a lot of fun into those thirty

years. But if that's not to be, then I'll just pack fun into whatever time I do have.

57

A Way to Understand Optimism

AFTER I learned I had cancer, one of my doctors gave me some advice. "It's important," he said, "to behave as if you're going to be around awhile."

I was already way ahead of him.

"Doc, I just bought a new convertible and got a vasectomy. What more do you want from me?"

Look, I'm not in denial about my situation. I am maintaining my clear-eyed sense of the inevitable. I'm living like I'm dying. But at the same time, I'm very much living like I'm still living.

Some oncologists' offices will schedule appointments for patients six months out. For the patients, it's an optimistic signal that the doctors expect them to live. There are terminally ill people who look at the doctor's appointment cards on their bulletin boards and say to themselves, "I'm going to make it to that. And when I get there, I'm going to get good news."

Herbert Zeh, my surgeon in Pittsburgh, says he worries about patients who are inappropriately optimistic or ill-informed. At the same time, he is upset when patients are told by friends and acquaintances that they have to be optimistic or their treatments won't work. It pains him to see patients who are having a tough day healthwise and assume it's because they weren't positive enough.

My personal take on optimism is that as a mental state, it can enable you to do tangible things to improve your physical state. If you're optimistic, you're better able to endure brutal chemo, or keep searching for late-breaking medical treatments.

Dr. Zeh calls me his poster boy for "the healthy balance between optimism and realism." He sees me trying to embrace my cancer as another life experience.

But I love that my vasectomy doubled as both appropriate birth control and an optimistic gesture about my future. I love driving around in my new convertible. I love thinking I might find a way to become the one-in-a-million guy who beats this late-stage cancer. Because even if I don't, it's a better mindset to help me get through each day.

58

The Input of Others

SINCE MY last lecture began spreading on the Internet, I've been hearing from so many people I've known over the years—from childhood neighbors to long-ago acquaintances. And I'm grateful for their warm words and thoughts.

It has been a delight to read notes from former students and colleagues. One coworker recalled advice I gave him when he was a non-tenured faculty member. He said I had warned him to pay attention to any and all comments made by department chairs. (He remembers me telling him: "When the chair casually suggests that perhaps you might consider doing something, you should visualize a cattle prod.") A former student emailed to say I had helped inspire him to create a new personal-development Web site titled "Stop Sucking and Live a Life of Abundance," designed to help people who are living far below their potential. That sounded sort of like my philosophy, though certainly not my exact words.

And just to keep things in perspective, from the "Some-Things-*Never*-Change" department, an unrequited crush from high school wrote to wish me well and gently reminded me why I was way too nerdy for her back then (also letting slip that she'd gone on to marry a *real* doctor).

More seriously, thousands of strangers also have written to me, and I've been buoyed by their good wishes. Many shared advice on how they and their loved ones have coped with matters of death and dying.

A woman who lost her forty-eight-year-old husband to pancreatic cancer said his "last speech" was to a small audience: her, his children, his parents and his siblings. He thanked them for their guidance and love, reminisced about the places he had gone with them, and told them what had mattered most to him in life. This woman said counseling had helped her family after her husband died: "Knowing what I know now, Mrs. Pausch and your children will have a need to talk, cry and remember."

Another woman, whose husband died of a brain tumor when their children were ages three and eight, offered insights for me to pass along to Jai. "You can survive the unimaginable," she wrote. "Your children will be a tremendous source of comfort and love, and will be the best reason to wake up every morning and smile."

She went on: "Take the help that's offered while Randy lives, so you can enjoy your time with him. Take the help that's offered when he's no longer here, so you can have the strength for what's important. Join others who have this kind of loss. They will be a comfort for you and your children." This woman suggested that Jai reassure our kids, as they get older, that they will have a normal life. There will be graduations, marriages, children of their own. "When a parent dies at such an early age, some children think that other normal life cycle events may not happen for them, either."

I heard from a man in his early forties with serious heart problems. He wrote to tell me about Krishnamurti, a spiritual leader in India who died in 1986. Krishnamurti was once asked what is the most appropriate thing to say to a friend who was about to die. He answered: "Tell your friend that in his death, a part of you dies and goes with him. Wherever he goes, you also go. He will not be alone." In his email to me, this man was reassuring: "I know you are not alone."

I have also been moved by comments and good wishes from some well-known people who got in touch as a result of the lecture. For instance, TV news anchor Diane Sawyer interviewed me, and when the cameras were off, helped me think more clearly about the touchstones I'll be leaving for my kids. She gave me an incredible piece of advice. I knew I was going to leave my kids letters and videos. But she told me the crucial thing is to tell them the specific idiosyncratic ways in which I related to them. So I've been thinking a lot about that. I've decided to tell each of my kids things like: "I love the way you tilted back your head when you laughed." I will give them specific stuff they can grasp.

And Dr. Reiss, the counselor Jai and I see, has helped me find strategies to avoid losing myself in the stress of my periodic cancer scans, so I'm able to focus on my family with an open heart, a positive outlook and almost of all my attention. I had spent much of my life doubting the effectiveness of counseling. Now, with my back against the wall, I see how hugely helpful it can be. I wish I could travel through oncology wards telling this to patients who are trying to tough it out on their own.

*   *   *

Many, many people have written to me about matters of faith. I've so appreciated their comments and their prayers.

I was raised by parents who believed that faith was something very personal. I didn't discuss my specific religion in my lecture because I wanted to talk about universal principles that apply to all faiths—to share things I had learned through my relationships with people.

Some of those relationships, of course, I have found at

church. M. R. Kelsey, a woman from our church, came and sat with me in the hospital every day for eleven days after my surgery. And since my diagnosis, my minister has been very helpful. We belonged to the same swimming pool in Pittsburgh, and the day after I'd learned my condition was terminal, we were both there. He was sitting by the pool and I climbed up on the diving board. I winked at him, then did a flip off the board.

When I got to the side of the pool, he said to me, "You seem to be the picture of good health, Randy." I told him: "That's the cognitive dissonance. I feel good and look great, but we heard yesterday that my cancer is back and the doctors say I only have three to six months."

He and I have since talked about the ways I might best prepare for death.

"You have life insurance, right?" he said.

"Yes, it's all in place," I told him.

"Well, you also need emotional insurance," he said. And then he explained that the premiums of emotional insurance would be paid for with my time, not my money.

To that end, he suggested that I needed to spend hours making videotapes of myself with the kids, so they'll have a record of how we played and laughed. Years from now, they will be able to see the ease with which we touched each other and interacted. He also gave me his thoughts on specific things I could do for Jai to leave her a record of my love.

"If you cover the premiums on your emotional insurance

now, while you're feeling OK, there will be less weighing on you in the months ahead," he said. "You'll be more at peace."

My friends. My loved ones. My minister. Total strangers. Every single day I receive input from people who wish me well and boost my spirits. I've truly gotten to see examples of the best in humanity, and I'm so grateful for that. I've never felt alone on this ride I'm taking.

VI

FINAL REMARKS

59

Dreams for My Children

THERE ARE so many things I want to tell my children, and right now, they're too young to understand. Dylan just turned six. Logan is three. Chloe is eighteen months old. I want the kids to know who I am, what I've always believed in, and all the ways in which I've come to love them. Given their ages, so much of this would be over their heads.

I wish the kids could understand how desperately I don't want to leave them.

Jai and I haven't even told them yet that I'm dying. We've been advised that we should wait until I'm more symptomatic. Right now, though I've been given just months to live, I still look pretty healthy. And so my kids remain unaware that in my every encounter with them I'm saying goodbye.

It pains me to think that when they're older, they won't have a father. When I cry in the shower, I'm not usually thinking, "I won't get to see them do this" or "I won't get to see them do that." I'm thinking about the kids not having a father. I'm focused more on what they're going to lose than on what I'm going to lose. Yes, a percentage of my sadness is, "I won't, I won't, I won't . . ." But a bigger part of me grieves for them. I keep thinking, "They won't . . . they won't . . . they won't." That's what chews me up inside, when I let it.

I know their memories of me may be fuzzy. That's why I'm trying to do things with them that they'll find unforgettable. I want their recollections to be as sharp as possible. Dylan and I went on a mini-vacation to swim with dolphins. A kid swims with dolphins, he doesn't easily forget it. We took lots of photos.

I'm going to bring Logan to Disney World, a place that I know he'll love as much as I do. He'd like to meet Mickey Mouse. I've met him, so I can make the introduction. Jai and I will bring Dylan along as well, since every experience Logan has these days doesn't seem complete unless he's engaged in the action with his big brother.

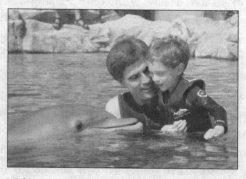

Making memories with Dylan.

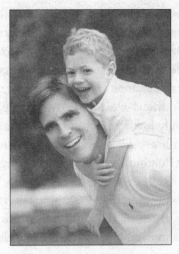

Logan, the ultimate Tigger.

Every night at bedtime, when I ask Logan to tell me the best part of his day, he always answers: "Playing with Dylan." When I ask him for the worst part of his day, he also answers: "Playing with Dylan." Suffice it to say, they're bonded as brothers.

I'm aware that Chloe may have no memory of me at all. She's too young. But I want her to grow up knowing that I was the first man ever to fall in love with her. I'd always thought the father/daughter thing was overstated. But I can tell you, it's real. Sometimes, she looks at me and I just become a puddle.

There are so many things Jai will be able to tell them about me when they're older. She might talk about my optimism, the way I embraced having fun, the high standards I tried to set in my life. She may diplomatically tell them some of the things that made me exasperating; my overly analytical approach to life, my insistence (too often) that I know best. But she's modest, much more modest than me, and she might not tell the kids this: that in our marriage, she had a guy who really deeply truly loved her. And she won't tell them all the sacrifices she made. Any mother of three small children is consumed with taking care of them. Throw in a cancer-stricken husband and the result is a woman who is always dealing with someone else's needs, not her own. I want my kids to know how selfless she was in caring for all of us.

Lately, I've been making a point of speaking to people who lost parents when they were very young. I want to know what got them through the hard times, and what keepsakes have been most meaningful to them.

They told me they found it consoling to learn about how much their mothers and fathers loved them. The more they knew, the more they could still feel that love.

They also wanted reasons to be proud; they wanted to believe that their parents were incredible people. Some of them sought specifics on their parents' accomplishments. Some chose to build myths. But all had yearnings to know what made their parents special.

These people told me something else, too. Since they have so few of their own memories of their parents, they found it reassuring to know that their parents died with great memories of them.

To that end, I want my kids to know that my memories of them fill my head.

Let's start with Dylan. I admire how loving and empathetic he is. If another child is hurt, Dylan will bring over a toy or blanket.

Another trait I see in Dylan: He's analytical, like his old man. He has already figured out that the questions are more important than the answers. A lot of kids ask, "Why? Why? Why?" One rule in our house is that you may not ask one-word questions. Dylan embraces that idea. He loves to formulate full-sentence questions, and his inquisitiveness goes beyond his years. I remember his pre-school teachers raving about him, telling us: "When you're with Dylan you find yourself thinking: I want to see what kind of adult this kid turns into."

Dylan is also the king of curiosity. Wherever he is, he's looking somewhere else and thinking, "Hey, there's something over there! Let's go look at it or touch it or take it apart." If there's a white picket fence, some kids will take a stick to it and walk along listening to the "thwack, thwack, thwack!" Dylan would go one better. He'd use the stick to pry one of the pickets loose, and then he'd use the picket to do the thwacking thing because it's thicker and sounds better.

For his part, Logan makes everything an adventure. When he was born, he got stuck in the birth canal. It took two doctors, pulling with forceps, to bring him into the world. I remember one of the doctors, his foot on the table, pulling with all his might. At one point the doctor turned to me and said:

"I've got chains and Clydesdales in the back if this doesn't work."

It was a tough passage for Logan. Given how cramped he was for so long in the birth canal, his arms weren't moving just after he was born. We were worried, but not for long. Once he started moving, he never really stopped. He's just this phenomenal ball of positive energy; completely physical and gregarious. When he smiles, he smiles with his whole face; he's the ultimate Tigger. He's also a kid who's up for everything and befriends everyone. He's only three years old, but I'm predicting he'll be the social chair of his college fraternity.

Chloe, meanwhile, is all girl. I say that with a bit of awe because until she came along, I couldn't fathom what that meant. She was scheduled to be a C-section baby, but Jai's water broke, and not long after we got to the hospital, Chloe just slipped out. (That's my description. Jai might say "slipped out" is a phrase only a man could come up with!) Anyway, for me, holding Chloe for the first time, looking into this tiny girl's face, well, it was one of the most intense and spiritual moments of my life. There was this connection I felt, and it was different from the one I had with the boys. I am now a member of the Wrapped Around My Daughter's Finger Club.

I love watching Chloe. Unlike Dylan and Logan, who are always so physically daring, Chloe is careful, maybe even dainty. We have a safety gate at the top of our staircase, but she doesn't really need it because all of her efforts go into not getting hurt. Having grown accustomed to two boys who rumble their way down any staircase, fearing no danger, this is a new experience for Jai and me.

I love all three of my kids completely and differently. And I want them to know that I will love them for as long as they live. I will.

Given my limited time, though, I've had to think about how I might reinforce my bonds with them. So I'm building separate lists of my memories of each of the kids. I'm making videos so they can see me talking about what they've meant to me. I'm writing letters to them. I also see the video of my last lecture—and this book, too—as pieces of myself that I can leave for them. I even have a large plastic bin filled with mail I received in the weeks after the lecture. Someday, the kids might want to look through that bin, and my hope is that they'll be pleased to find both friends and strangers who had found the talk meaningful.

Because I've been so vocal about the power of childhood dreams, some people have been asking lately about the dreams I have for my children.

I have a direct answer for that.

It can be a very disruptive thing for parents to have specific dreams for their kids. As a professor, I've seen many unhappy college freshman picking majors that are all wrong for them. Their parents have put them on a train, and too often, judging by the crying during my office hours, the result is a train wreck.

As I see it, a parent's job is to encourage kids to develop a joy for life and a great urge to follow their own dreams. The best we can do is to help them develop a personal set of tools for the task.

So my dreams for my kids are very exact: I want them to find their own path to fulfillment. And given that I won't be there, I want to make this clear: Kids, don't try to figure out what I wanted you to become. I want you to become what *you* want to become.

Having seen so many students go through my classrooms, I've come to know that a lot of parents don't realize the power of their words. Depending on a child's age and sense of self, an offhand comment from Mom or Dad can feel like a shove from a bulldozer. I'm not even sure I should have made the reference to Logan growing up to be social chair of a fraternity. I don't want him to end up in college thinking that I expected him to join a fraternity, or to be a leader there—or anything. His life will be his life. I would just urge my kids to find their way with enthusiasm and passion. And I want them to feel as if I am there with them, whatever path they choose.

60

Jai and Me

_____

As any family dealing with cancer knows, caregivers are often pushed to the sidelines. Patients get to focus on themselves. They're the objects of adulation and sympathy. Caregivers do the heavy lifting, with little time to deal with their own pain and grief.

My wife, Jai, is a cancer caregiver with even more on her plate: three little kids. So as I prepared to give my last lecture, I made a decision. If this talk was to be my moment, I wanted some way to show everyone how much I love and appreciate her.

It happened like this: Near the end of the lecture, as I reviewed the lessons I'd learned in my life, I mentioned how vital it is to focus on other people, not just yourself. Looking offstage, I asked: "Do we have a concrete example of focusing on somebody else over there? Could we bring it out?"

Because the day before had been Jai's birthday, I arranged to have a large birthday cake with a single candle waiting on a rolling table offstage. As the cake was wheeled out by Jai's friend Cleah Schlueter, I explained to the audience that I hadn't given Jai a proper birthday, and thought it might be nice if I could get four hundred people to sing to her. They applauded the idea and began singing.

"Happy birthday to you. Happy birthday to you . . ."

Realizing some might not know her name, I quickly said, "Her name is Jai . . ."

"Happy birthday, dear Jai . . ."

It was so wonderful. Even people in the nearby overflow room, watching the lecture on a video screen, were singing.

As we all sang, I finally allowed myself to look at Jai. She sat in her front-row seat, wiping away tears with this surprised smile on her face, looking so lovely—bashful and beautiful, pleased and overwhelmed. . . .

There are so many things Jai and I are discussing as we work to come to terms with what her life will be like after I'm gone. "Lucky" is a strange word to use to describe my situation, but a part of me does feel fortunate that I didn't get hit by the proverbial bus. Cancer has given me the time to have these vital conversations with Jai that wouldn't be possible if my fate were a heart attack or a car accident.

What are we talking about?

For starters, we both try to remember that some of the best caregiving advice we've ever heard comes from flight attendants: "Put on your own oxygen mask before assisting others." Jai is such a giver that she often forgets to take care of herself. When we become physically or emotionally run down, we can't help anybody else, least of all small children.

So there's nothing weak or selfish about taking some fraction of your day to be alone, recharging your batteries. In my experience as a parent, I've found it hard to recharge in the presence of small children. Jai knows that she'll have to give herself permission to make herself a priority.

I've also reminded her that she's going to make mistakes, and to just accept that. If I were able to live, we'd be making those mistakes together. Mistakes are part of the process of parenting, and she shouldn't attribute them all to the fact that she'll be raising the kids herself.

Some single parents fall into the trap of trying to compensate by giving the kids material things. Jai knows: No material possessions can make up for a missing parent, and they can actually do harm in establishing a kid's values.

It's possible that Jai, like many parents, will find the most challenging years to be when the kids become teenagers. Having been around students all my life, I'd like to think I would come into my own as a father of teens. I'd be tough, but I'd understand the mind-set. So I'm sorry I won't be there to help Jai when the time comes.

The good news, though, is that other people—friends and family—will also want to help, and Jai plans to let them. All children need a fabric of people in their lives who love them, and that's especially true for kids who've lost a parent. I think back to my own parents. They knew they couldn't be the only crucial influences in my life. That's why my dad signed me up to play football with Jim Graham. Jai will be on the lookout for some Coach Grahams for our kids.

As for the obvious question, well, here's my answer:

Most of all, I want Jai to be happy in the years ahead. So if she finds happiness through remarriage, that will be great. If she finds happiness without remarrying, that also will be great.

Jai and I work hard at our marriage. We've gotten so much better at communicating, at sensing each other's needs and strengths, and at finding more things to love about each other. So it saddens us that we won't get to experience this richness in our marriage for the next thirty or forty years. We won't get to amortize the hard efforts we've put in so far. Still, we wouldn't trade our eight years of marriage for anything.

I know that so far, I've been handling my diagnosis pretty well. Jai has, too. As she says: "No one needs to cry for me." She means it. But we want to be honest, too. Though counseling has helped tremendously, we've had some tough times. We've cried together in bed, fallen back asleep, woken up and cried some more. We've gotten through in part by focusing on the tasks at hand. We can't fall to pieces. We've got to get some sleep, because one of us has to get up in the morning and give the kids breakfast. That person, for the record, is almost always Jai.

I recently celebrated my forty-seventh birthday, and Jai had to wrestle with the question: "What do you get the man you love for his last birthday?" She opted for a watch and a big-screen TV. Though I'm not a fan of TV—it's mankind's greatest time-waster—the gift was completely appropriate, since I'll be in bed so much at the end. TV will be one of my last links to the outside world.

There are days when Jai tells me things and there's little I can say in response. She has told me: "I can't imagine rolling over in bed and you're not there." And: "I can't picture myself taking the kids on vacation and you not being with us." And: "Randy, you're always the planner. Who's going to make the plans?"

I'm not worried. Jai will make the plans just fine.

*   *   *

I really had no idea what I would do or say after the audience sang "Happy Birthday" to Jai. But as I urged her onto the stage, and she came toward me, a natural impulse overtook me. Her, too, I guess. We embraced and we kissed, first on the lips, and then I kissed her cheek. The crowd kept applauding. We heard them, but it was like they were miles away.

As we held each other, Jai whispered something in my ear.

"Please don't die."

It sounds like Hollywood dialogue. But that's what she said. I just hugged her more tightly.

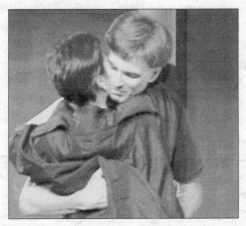

61

The Dreams Will Come to You

F OR DAYS, I had worried that I'd be unable to get through the final lines of my lecture without choking up. So I had a contingency plan. I placed the last few sentences of the talk on four slides. If, in the moment on stage, I couldn't bring myself to say the words, my plan was to click silently through the slides, and then simply say "Thank you for coming today."

I had been on stage for just over an hour. Given the chemo side effects, the long stretch on my feet, and the emotions involved, I was truly feeling spent.

At the same time, I felt at peace and fulfilled. My life had come full circle. I had first made the list of my childhood dreams when I was eight years old. Now, thirty-eight years later, that very list had helped me say what I needed to say and carried me through.

Many cancer patients say their illness gives them a new and deeper appreciation for life. Some even say they are grateful for their disease. I have no such gratitude for my cancer, although I'm certainly grateful for having advance notice of my death. In addition to allowing me to prepare my family for the future, that time gave me the chance to go to Carnegie Mellon and give my last lecture. In a sense, it allowed me to "leave the field under my own power."

And my list of childhood dreams had continued to serve so many purposes. Without it, who knows if I would have been able to thank all the people who deserved my thanks. Ultimately, that little list had allowed me to say goodbye to those who meant so much to me.

There's something else. As a high-tech guy, I never fully understood the artists and actors I've known and taught over the years. They would sometimes talk about the things inside them that "needed to come out." I thought that sounded self-indulgent. I should have been more empathetic. My hour on stage had taught me something. (At least I was still learning!) I did have things inside me that desperately needed to come out. I didn't give the lecture just because I *wanted* to. I gave the lecture because I had to.

I also knew why my closing lines would be so emotional for me. It was because the end of the talk had to be a distillation of how I felt about the end of my life.

As I wound down, I had taken a minute to review some of the key points of the lecture. And then I offered a summation, but with a twist; a surprise ending, if you will.

"So today's talk was about achieving childhood dreams," I said. "But did you figure out the head fake?"

I paused. The room was quiet.

"It's not about how to achieve your dreams. It's about how

to lead your life. If you lead your life the right way, the karma will take care of itself. The dreams will come to you."

I clicked to the next slide, and a question filled the large screen: "Have you figured out the second head fake?"

I took a breath. I decided to speak at a slightly faster clip than I had before. Maybe if I just talked faster, I thought, I could get through it. I repeated the words on screen.

"Have you figured out the second head fake?"

Then I told them: The talk wasn't just for those in the room. "It was for my kids."

I clicked to the very last slide, a photo of me standing by our swing set, holding a smiling Logan with my right arm and sweet Chloe with my left, Dylan sitting happily on my shoulders.

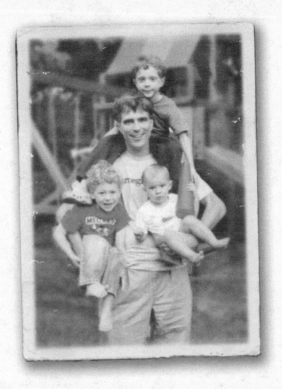

Randy Pausch was a professor of Computer Science, Human Computer Interaction, and Design at Carnegie Mellon University. From 1988 to 1997, he taught at the University of Virginia. He was an award-winning teacher and researcher, and worked with Adobe, Google, Electronic Arts (EA), and Walt Disney Imagineering, and pioneered the non-profit Alice project. He lived in Virginia with his wife and three children. Randy lost his battle with pancreatic cancer on July 25th, 2008.

I was trying to put myself in a bottle that would one day wash up on the beach for my children. If I were a painter, I would have painted for them. But I am a lecturer, so I lectured.

Acknowledgments

M<small>Y GREAT</small> thanks to Bob Miller, David Black, and Gary Morris. I wish to especially thank our editor, Will Balliett, for his great kindness and integrity throughout, and Jeffrey Zaslow, for his incredible talent and professionalism.

* * *

The full set of people I must thank will not fit on this page. Fortunately, web pages scroll: please visit **www.thelastlecture.com** for a full list of acknowledgments and attributions. Video of my "last lecture" can also be viewed from that site.

* * *

My life will be lost to pancreatic cancer. Two organizations I have worked with that are dedicated to fighting this disease are:

The Pancreatic Cancer Action Network
www.pancan.org

The Lustgarten Foundation
www.lustgarten.org